TYPE 2

ALSO BY

MIRYAM EHRLICH WILLIAMSON

Blood Sugar Blues
The Fibromyalgia Relief Book
Fibromyalgia: A Comprehensive Approach

TYPE 2

A BOOK OF SUPPORT FOR TYPE 2 DIABETICS

Miryam Ehrlich Williamson

Walker & Company
New York

First published in the United States of America in 2003 by Walker Publishing Company, Inc.

Published simultaneously in Canada by Fitzhenry and Whiteside, Markham, Ontario L3R 4T8

Medical disclaimer: The treatments and therapies described in this book are not intended to replace the services of a trained health professional. Your own physical condition may require specific modifications or precautions. Before undertaking any treatment or therapy, you should consult your physician or health care provider. Any application of the ideas, suggestions, and procedures set forth in this book are at the reader's discretion.

For information about permission to reproduce selections from this book, write to Permissions, Walker & Company, 435 Hudson Street, New York, New York 10014

Library of Congress Cataloging-in Publication Data

Williamson, Miryam Ehrlich.
Type 2 : a book of support for type 2 diabetics / Miryam Ehrlich Williamson.
p. cm.
Includes bibliographical references and index.
ISBN 0-8027-7666-3 (hbk. : alk. paper)
1. Noninsulin-dependent diabetes—Popular works.
I. Title: Type two. II. Title.

RC662.18.W557 2003
616.4'62—dc21 2003042257

Book design by M. J. DiMassi

Visit Walker & Company's Web site at www.walkerbooks.com

Printed in the United States of America
2 4 6 8 10 9 7 5 3 1

TO LINDA

CONTENTS

Acknowledgments xi
Introduction 1

1. Getting the Word 8
    Diagnosis Stories 10
    Reactions to the News 17

2. Settling In 24
    What the Doctor Said 25
    The Road to Acceptance 33
    Beyond Acceptance 52

3. Learning the Ropes 56
    Getting the Information You Need 58
    Eating Right 63
    Testing 77
    Exercise 87

4. Jumping the Hurdles 97
    Standing Up for Yourself 97

Obstacles to Exercising and Losing Weight 102
Learning to Eat Again 105
Dealing with Complications 110
Interpersonal Relationships 116
Diabetes at Work 125
Testing in Public 129

5. Compulsive Overeating 132
Changing How You Think About Food 136
Overcoming Overeating with the OO Program 138
Making Peace with Food 148

6. Sexual Dysfunction 153
Not for Men Only 154
Not for Women Only 163
The Importance of Sex 167

7. From Struggle to Success 170
Attitude Is Everything 173
Knowledge Is Power 176
Words of Inspiration 180

Epilogue: What Lies Ahead 185

Glossary 191

Appendix 1. Internet Resources 197

Appendix 2. Oral Diabetes Medications and Their Actions and Side Effects 205

Appendix 3. Blood Glucose Monitors 213

Appendix 4. Additional Resources 219

Index 223

ACKNOWLEDGMENTS

More than a hundred people allowed me to interview them, generously sharing their time, thoughts, and feelings with me as I prepared this book. I learned from them all; their spirit and determination inspired me. The stories of many of these people appear here, their names changed to protect their privacy. I especially want to thank Julia Klaristenfeld, M.A., a talented psychotherapist, who read portions of the manuscript with sensitivity and insight. Jacqueline Johnson, my editor for the fourth time, was once again thorough and gentle in offering her suggestions. Jenny Bent, my agent, and Ed Hawes, my husband and best friend, were there without fail when I needed them. And without George Gibson's idea to begin with, this book would never have been written. To all who helped in this effort, I give my heartfelt thanks.

TYPE 2

INTRODUCTION

Gary reached into the shopping bag he had brought with him to the diabetes support group he was addressing. When he drew out the trousers he had worn to his godson's christening four years earlier, people gasped. Fully clothed, he stepped into the pants and held out the waistband at arm's length. A couple of men could have joined him in there. When he talked about how he had gone from massive to slim, from being in a diabetic coma to being a Type 2 diabetic who controlled his condition with diet and exercise, people began to think that maybe they could do a better job of taking care of themselves.

Maria, a registered Seneca Indian from the Six Nations Reserve in Ontario, watched her father and her maternal grandmother lose feet and legs to uncontrolled diabetes. During two pregnancies she herself developed gestational diabetes before being diagnosed with Type 2. Today Maria keeps her diabetes in check through diet and physical activities. She is hopeful that she'll never need medication or follow the path of her relatives in the downward spiral that is uncontrolled diabetes.

Vicki struggled with a lifelong compulsion to overeat that made it doubly difficult to control her diabetes. The more she denied herself the foods that made her blood sugar rise to dangerous levels, the more she found herself binge-eating those very foods. Vicki eventually stopped that vicious cycle by using a combination of insulin, oral medication, and a program designed to help her control her eating disorder. She is pleased with her progress and optimistic about her ability to improve her health.

Diabetes is a disease in which your body can't obtain energy from the food you eat. Normally, your digestive processes turn much of your food into glucose (sugar), which is absorbed into your blood. When glucose enters the bloodstream, a signal tells the pancreas to release insulin into the blood. Insulin unlocks your body's cells, allowing glucose that is not needed immediately to be stored for future use as energy. Diabetes is a disturbance of this process.

In Type 1 diabetes, the immune system attacks

the insulin-producing cells of the pancreas, destroying them and preventing new ones from taking their place. Eventually, the pancreas loses its ability to create insulin. When this happens, Type 1 diabetics must take insulin by injection. Most Type 1 diabetics develop the disease in childhood or early adulthood. Only about 5 percent of all diabetics have Type 1.

Most people with Type 2 diabetes are insulin resistant. While they produce enough insulin, their cells don't use it efficiently. Instead of being stored in the cells as energy, glucose is stored as fat, giving rise to obesity and the problems associated with high levels of fats in the blood: high cholesterol, high blood pressure, heart disease, and stroke. Some Type 2 diabetics are insulin deficient. The pancreas makes insulin, but not enough. These are the people known as *lean diabetics.* Unlike most Type 2s, they are not overweight. A few people with Type 2 diabetes have a combination of both disorders: They don't make enough insulin, and what they do make doesn't work the way it should.

The spread of Type 2 diabetes has taken on the characteristics of an epidemic, although the disease does not spread from person to person the way epidemic diseases usually do. According to the U.S. Centers for Disease Control, there was a

49 percent increase between 1990 and 2000 in the number of Americans who have diabetes. Between 1999 and 2000 alone, the incidence of Type 2 diabetes increased from 6.9 percent to 7.3 percent in the U.S. population. Type 2 diabetes used to be called *adult onset diabetes,* as opposed to Type 1, or *juvenile diabetes.* Now children are also developing the Type 2 variety. Experts relate its increasing occurrence in children to their decreasing physical activity. Many children today spend their spare time playing computer games and watching television, instead of playing outdoors. This sedentary lifestyle, coupled with the inevitable snacking that accompanies it, leads to obesity and insulin resistance at a younger age than ever before.

What makes diabetes so potentially serious an illness is that excessive sugar in the blood eventually leads to damage to nerve and blood vessel tissues. Thus, uncontrolled diabetes—chronically high blood sugar levels—can cause *diabetic neuropathy* (pain, numbness, and tingling) in hands and feet, damage to other crucial nerves, to kidneys, eyes, and the brain. Some of these attendant problems can be truly horrible, but the good news is that diabetes control is within your power. You don't have to give up and let it take over. That's what this book is about.

If you're reeling from the news that you have Type 2 diabetes and wondering how much it will alter your way of life, or if you've lived with the Type 2 diagnosis for some time now without ever really feeling in control, this book will help you. It profiles the struggles and successes of people in middle age, most of them between the ages of 40 and 60, who were diagnosed within the last few years and who had a tough time adjusting to the diagnosis and finding their way to controlling their diabetes. Their generosity in sharing the most intimate details of their lives makes this book a kind of personal support group for those who read it. People in diabetes support groups are often remarkably frank with one another, drawing knowledge and inspiration from the collective wisdom of those who are meeting similar challenges.

This book will help you understand your own reactions and feelings. It will give you new ideas about how to deal successfully with your condition. Like a good support group, this book will help you come to terms with diabetes's demands and learn to adjust to its requirements. You'll even learn why some Type 2s think diabetes has had a positive effect on their lives.

You will also learn that there are various approaches to managing Type 2 diabetes; that different strategies work for different people; and that, with patience and persistence, you can find your own way. You'll get to compare symptoms, experiences, and feelings. You'll learn that you're far from alone in your struggle—some 16 million people in the United States alone, 2 million in Canada, and millions more in other parts of the industrialized world, share your disease. You won't find here a bunch of starry-eyed Pollyannas. You'll read of complaints and regrets. But you'll never meet a more life-embracing group of people, and you're sure to learn something of value from each of them.

You will see the variety of circumstances that led people to their diagnosis, the multitude of symptoms—and sometimes the total lack of symptoms—that preceded diagnosis; the different reactions of individuals to the news that they have diabetes; the stages people went through before they accepted their situation; and where they wound up, physically and emotionally, after the initial news sank in. Seeing what others went through will validate your own feelings about having Type 2 diabetes.

Coping with diabetes requires problem solving and navigating many obstacles to spontaneity in one's daily life—from frequent blood sugar testing to rigorous meal planning. But there are several less obvious ways people have to adjust to the impact of diabetes on their lives, including sexual dysfunction.

Highlighting individual differences, this book covers a range of philosophies and specific actions that have helped others adapt to a chronic disease that can be inconvenient and sometimes downright dangerous. Also included is a discussion of self-advocacy—standing up for yourself in the face of indifferent or incompetent medical care. The tradition of seeing doctors as authority figures is so ingrained in some of us that it's hard to advocate for ourselves, but sometimes that's exactly what you must do if you're not satisfied with the care you're receiving.

At the back of the book you'll find a glossary of diabetes terms and several appendixes. The latter provide lists of helpful resources, as well as more details on oral medications and blood glucose monitors.

Imagine as you turn the page that you are entering a room where people much like you are seated in a circle, waiting to tell their stories. They've saved you a seat. Your support group meeting is about to begin.

1

GETTING THE WORD

Sit with a group of diabetics for a while, and you hear a range of diagnosis stories. Some people saw the doctor because they recognized diabetes's symptoms and expected to hear what they ultimately were told. Others went in for an entirely different reason and were shocked to learn what was really wrong. For some, the news came in the course of a routine physical examination; for others, it followed a crisis. Some have seen family members struggle with—or ignore—the disease and then fall prey themselves to the genetic tendency that often makes diabetes a family affair. Some have heard that obesity can lead to diabetes and were not in the least surprised when it caught up with them. To others, the slim ones who follow healthy eating guidelines and are physically active, the diagnosis may have come as a bitter shock.

TYPE 2

The magazine articles and Internet Web pages that tell you to watch out for diabetes symptoms tell only part of the story. To be sure, there is a constellation of symptoms—what you experience and report to the doctor—that almost always means diabetes. Most common among them are a thirst that no amount of fluids will quench and, consequently, the almost constant need to urinate. Another telling symptom is feeling tired most of the time—because of the inefficient conversion of food to energy. The doctor who hears these complaints should immediately think of diabetes and confirm it by looking for its primary sign: a high level of glucose (sugar) in the blood, sometimes called *hyperglycemia. Hyper-* means "too much," *-glyc-* refers to glucose, and *-emia* refers to the blood.

The Cecil Textbook of Medicine, a standard medical reference book, says a blood glucose reading higher than 200 mg/dl (milligrams of glucose per two-tenths of a pint of blood), taken without regard to the time of the most recent meal, is sufficient for a diabetes diagnosis, and that further tests only delay the start of treatment. Some physicians want to see the result of a fasting blood sugar test, the blood drawn at least twelve hours after the last time you had anything to eat, before giving a definitive diagnosis. A fasting blood sugar reading higher than 120 (some experts say 115) is reason to suspect diabetes. One over 140 makes it a sure thing.

DIAGNOSIS STORIES

Sometimes people can go to the doctor practically wearing a sign that says "I have diabetes" and come away without a diagnosis. Fifty-two-year-old Gary thinks he weighed more than 400 pounds when he went for a routine physical and complained of thirst, frequent urination, and lack of energy. He's not sure of his weight because the doctor's scale stopped at 350 pounds. Gary quotes his doctor as saying, "'Gee, your sugar level is getting up there.' I had never heard of a sugar level," he says. "My doctor said, 'You've got to watch your sugars.' I didn't know what he was talking about, so I started reading package labels, but I didn't know what was high and what was low. So I tried to avoid anything that had sugar in it, which is nearly impossible."

Over the next three months, Gary saw his doctor repeatedly—complaining mainly of overwhelming fatigue—but received no instructions on how to control his blood sugar until he landed in the hospital for five days. That was four years ago. Today Gary is hundreds of pounds lighter and keeps his condition in check. As a frequent speaker at meetings of diabetes support groups, he inspires others with his success story.

For Vernon, a forty-eight-year-old software engineer, diagnosis came as a doctor's offhand remark. Vernon had been troubled on and off for several years with an irregular heartbeat. Feeling particularly poorly, he went to his doctor, who told him, "Your diabetes is acting up." "I'm not diabetic," Vernon replied. "You are now," his doctor said.

When Greg, then fifty-one, showed up at his doctor's office complaining of unbearable thirst, a nearly constant urge to urinate, and fatigue, his doctor almost certainly knew what the diagnosis would be. I was "half dead, too tired to move," Greg recalls. The doctor did a blood glucose test on the spot. The test showed a blood sugar level of 670, more than three times the diagnostic level. Greg's doctor admitted him to the hospital immediately.

A very dry mouth, but not what she identified as thirst, troubled Helen, a fifty-five-year-old freelance writer. She was losing weight at a rapid pace and had recurring vaginal yeast infections. "I mentioned these symptoms individually to my internist over a period of a few months, but as isolated symptoms," she says. Helen didn't fit the classic diabetes profile. She wasn't overweight, and the disease didn't show up in her family history. She diagnosed herself using a guide to health that she had at home and trusted. "It apparently didn't occur to my doctor to put the symptoms together, but it occurred to me, and I told him so." The doctor doubted she had diabetes but tested her anyway. Her blood glucose level turned out to be 440.

Serena also diagnosed herself. At the time, she was a forty-four-year-old homemaker living in British Columbia, Canada. "[I was feeling] dizzy, sick to my stomach, thirsty all the time, and running to the bathroom," she recalls. She used a friend's glucose monitor, then consulted her doctor. In a series of tests, Serena's blood glucose readings ranged from 13.5 to 18.9. Canadians do not report blood glucose levels the same way that Americans do. According to the Canadian Diabetes Association, multiplying a given Canadian measurement by 18.2 gives you the U.S. equivalent, which means that Serena's blood sugar levels were between 246 and 344 at the time she was diagnosed.

Some medicines, whether prescription or over the counter, can mask diabetes's symptoms, delaying the diagnosis and giving the disease more of a chance to do damage. Roberta, a forty-nine-year-old retired nurse, thought her continual need to urinate was caused by the diuretic she was taking to fight tissue swelling (a little-recognized sign of insulin resistance, a leading cause of Type 2 diabetes). Alana, a thirty-seven-year-old emergency medical technician, blamed her constant thirst on allergies and the antihistamines and decongestants she took to relieve the symptoms. She thought thirst was a family characteristic. Older relatives told her, "We're a dry family. We just always stay dried out," she says. Roberta and Alana are Native Americans, members of a group with a particularly high incidence of Type 2 diabetes.

Blurry vision is another symptom that often accompanies diabetes. When Marcia realized that cleaning her glasses wasn't going to help her see any better, the fifty-one-year-old administrative secretary checked with her doctor. Her blood glucose reading was 181. Her doctor didn't wait for a second test to start treating her for diabetes.

Robert, an electronics technician, was fifty-seven when he suddenly started experiencing the classic nonstop thirst, an incessant urge to urinate, and an unexplained weight loss. But he knew nothing about diabetes and didn't recognize the danger signs. So he was stunned when he went in for his yearly physical and received the news that his blood sugar level was 350 and that he had diabetes.

For some, the symptoms that precede diagnosis are more dramatic than thirst, frequent urination, fatigue, and weight loss. At fifty-four, Raymond was starting a second career as a psychotherapist when he went to a neurologist with neck pain. "I was paralyzed with pain for about a month. It took me nearly two hours to complete a thirty-minute drive to work because every few minutes I'd have to pull over and stop to stretch and deal with the pain," he remembers. The neurologist wrote in his report that diabetes-induced nerve damage could be the cause of Raymond's pain. When Raymond had a fasting blood sugar test, the reading was 360. After his diagnosis, Raymond learned that depression, which he had been fighting for years, can often precede diabetes by as much as ten years. There's no way to tell whether the stress that accompanies depression precipitates the diabetes, or vice versa. Raymond says, "It is the chicken-and-egg thing. No one is willing to say that if you get depressed, it will cause diabetes—or if you have diabetes, it will cause depression. But the two frequently go hand in hand."

Paul, a fifty-four-year-old postal service worker, saw his doctor after getting dizzy and falling off his motorcycle. He was knocked unconscious but didn't break any bones. It wasn't Paul's first bout with dizziness, but it was the most life-threatening. Suspecting reactive hypoglycemia, a condition that often precedes diabetes, the doctor did a finger stick, tested Paul's blood glucose level, and immediately gave him an insulin shot. "I asked why, and he said I was diabetic. My blood sugar was over 450," he says, adding, "I'd had lots of thirst, but I wasn't big on sweets, so diabetes never entered my mind. I didn't know then that, for me, a pile of rice is just as bad as a piece of cake."

Charles, a forty-seven-year-old telecommunications analyst, went to a walk-in clinic for treatment of a gastrointestinal virus. The doctor told him his blood sugar level was 350. "It was a total surprise," Charles says. Later, he realized he'd been having classic diabetic symptoms for about five years. "I hadn't considered it strange that my feet were turning brown," he says wryly.

Thad, a fifty-three-year-old insurance claims examiner, didn't fit the diabetes pattern at all. Thad is the second oldest in a family of eight siblings. His brother Greg, fifteen months older than Thad, was diagnosed with Type 2 diabetes at forty-two. Heavier and less physically active, Greg didn't pay much attention to his health while Thad, who wasn't overweight, ran twenty miles a week and lifted weights. After twelve years of uncontrolled diabetes, Greg died unexpectedly. "He went to sleep and just didn't wake up," Thad says. "His heart had just given out. No pain for him, anyway."

Even though he was aware of the relationship between lifestyle choices and diabetes, his closeness to his brother, both emotionally and in terms of age, led Thad to call his family doctor. "I was feeling great and didn't have any symptoms," Thad recalls. The doctor did a complete physical checkup. Readings above 180 on two successive blood sugar tests led the doctor to diagnose diabetes. Disbelieving, Thad nevertheless took the prescribed medicine, which reduced the amount of glucose his liver produced, and gave up sweets. "Although I had a sweet tooth, I could give up sweets because I figured they would be poison to me," he says. He thought the doctor was being an alarmist, and that if he eliminated sugar from his diet he'd be home free. He wasn't. After a dinner of meat loaf and mashed potatoes, his glucose meter reading was 222—higher than the readings that led to his diagnosis. "That scared me. I decided maybe the doctor was right," he says.

REACTIONS TO THE NEWS

Just as they vary in symptoms and the circumstances under which they are diagnosed, people with Type 2 diabetes differ widely in the way they react to the news. Many are understandably shocked or dismayed at the news that they have an incurable illness. Some feel overwhelmed; others take a fatalistic attitude, often because the disease runs in their family and they've been expecting it to strike them. Often, those who have lost a loved one to diabetes are terrified, fearing a similar fate. Individual reactions can run the gamut from anger, resentment, and disbelief to resignation, determination, and even relief.

Even though she'd been expecting it, the emotional impact of the words *you have diabetes* came as a shock to Elaine, fifty-two, who used to work in international sales and marketing. It was four months since her mother had died of kidney failure resulting from poorly controlled diabetes ("Her choice," Elaine says). Images of her mother, nearly blind and with poor circulation in her legs, came to her mind when she heard her own diagnosis. "I was pretty scared, even though realistically I knew that did not have to be my fate," Elaine says.

Shortly after Rose's mother died of complications of uncontrolled diabetes, this forty-four-year-old registered nurse used her mother's glucose monitor to test her own blood. "Diabetes is everywhere in my family, so I would have been more than aware of any excessive thirst or urination. There was nothing like that, no sores that would not heal, none of the normal warning signs," she says. "I would say that fatigue and a never-ending slight headache had been my only symptoms. Since my mom had died unexpectedly only a month before, I thought the fatigue was part of the grieving process." Rose's blood glucose level was 225. "I woke up my husband and tested his blood sugar. It was 96. I cried for an hour," she recalls. "It was only after my sugars were under control, three months later, that I realized how badly I had been feeling."

A family history of diabetes didn't help Roberta, the retired nurse, accept the news that her blood sugar level was over 300. The doctor told her to make an appointment for another test in two weeks. "I panicked," she says. "I felt like I'd just heard a death sentence. Both grandparents on my father's side died from diabetes. Aunts and uncles have passed away also. I'd seen them undergo amputations and watched most of them go blind." In the first hours after she received her diagnosis, Roberta says she saw her life draining away. Today, though, she says, "I am not going down without a fight."

Like Roberta, Grace, a forty-nine-year-old accounting clerk, was terrified when she was rushed to the hospital, too weak to stand up, and learned her blood glucose level was 575. She had never heard of diabetes before her diagnosis. She had no idea what the word meant, nor did she know that her African-American heredity put her at higher risk for the disease. Even the classic warning signs of excessive thirst, frequent urination, and sudden weight loss—all of which she had experienced—meant nothing to her. She decided to prepare herself to die.

Vernon greeted his diagnosis with "shock, disbelief, dismay, and denial." He says it took him several years to accept that he had diabetes and get on with learning to control it.

Thad, whose brother had recently died of diabetes complications, was resentful. "I felt that it wasn't fair," he says, "the way someone who had never smoked but got lung cancer anyway might feel. I had a supervisor at the time who was shorter than I was and weighed 320 pounds, but he didn't have diabetes. Three quarters of the people with diabetes are obese, and I wasn't even overweight!"

Ross, a fifty-one-year-old certified accountant, was also angry because he had no warning. As far as he knows, he is the first in his family to become diabetic. His response was to learn all he could by joining the Canadian Diabetes Association in his Canadian province, where he now serves on the board of directors.

Marissa, a forty-eight-year-old secretary at a major medical center, whose diabetes showed up in the aftermath of a gallbladder operation, found herself thinking that if she lost weight she would "lose the diagnosis," she says. For a while she was overwhelmed with the details of managing the disease.

Carl, a social worker in Australia, denied the fact of his disease for a brief period, knowing that he must take control but feeling the need to give himself time to come to terms with the situation.

Rand, a writer who is fifty-six, greeted his diagnosis with relief, because it explained years of overwhelming fatigue and heavy sweating.

Delores, retired at forty-seven, always had her blood sugar checked when she saw her primary care physician for other reasons, and she always passed the test. Then, a few weeks after her father died of diabetes complications, her blood sugar level was 189 three and a half hours after her last meal. "You're diabetic—no ifs, ands, or buts," the doctor told her. She wasn't surprised. When the doctor told her to cut her food intake in half to lose weight, Delores told him that wasn't at all realistic. She decided to learn everything she could about getting her blood sugar under control, and only after she'd done that would she try to lose weight.

For Barbara, fifty, who works as a mental health associate, the moment of truth came during a physical exam when she was hired for a new job. A blood test showed a fasting blood sugar level of more than 220. The doctor told her to see a dietician at the local hospital, stay away from sugar, and lose some weight. She recalls her reaction: "[I decided to] skip the dietician. I've tried more diets than I care to admit and never succeeded, so why put myself through it all over again?" For the next few months she tried to suppress her fear. "Then," she says, "I got curious, and tired of feeling helpless and scared, and I started seeking information."

Daniel, a fifty-eight-year-old economist, wasn't particularly concerned when, during a routine checkup, his doctor told him his blood glucose level of 135 suggested "incipient diabetes." He greeted the news with a combination of "interest, skepticism, and mild concern." The doctor gave him a prescription for an oral medication and told him to modify his diet. "It seemed like biblically just retribution for years of weight gain and a sedentary lifestyle," Daniel says. But it took another couple of years before he was ready to change his eating habits.

Greg greeted his diagnosis with two words: *no way!* But before long, he says, his attitude changed. "I decided I can work with this. It won't rule my life, but I will live with it."

Raymond also took his diagnosis as a challenge. "I know that most people get shocked and depressed and bummed out and scared," he says, "but my reaction was different. When my second fasting glucose came in at 360, my doctor said, 'That makes it official. You are diabetic.' And I grinned from ear to ear, and said, 'This is going to be fun.' The doctor's jaw dropped. He said, 'What on earth do you mean?'"

Raymond says he knew most of his life he'd wind up with diabetes. Both his parents had the disease. When Raymond was a child, his father, a physician, had the entire family on a low-carbohydrate, high-protein diet, meant to stave off the disease. Even so, Raymond says, he was always overweight. He received his diagnosis within a few months of the age his father was when he was diagnosed. Raymond told the doctor, "Whatever it takes—medication, diet, exercise—I'm going to control this. I know that if my glucose levels stay out of control, you're going to cut off my feet, I'm going to go blind, and I'm going to be impotent—and if I lose my feet and go blind, the last thing I want in the world is to be impotent because I'll have nothing else to do."

Raymond isn't the only one to greet his diagnosis with humor. Norm, a sixty-one-year-old author and columnist, says his initial reaction was to accept the idea without dismay. The day after he received his diagnosis, Norm read an article in the *New York Times* about Type 2 diabetes. He recalls: "[Upon learning that] it was the hot new disease among people my age, I thought, 'I'm so cool!'"

Rose, the nurse who diagnosed herself using her mother's glucose meter, soon stopped crying and declared, "Life changes now." Then she put on her workout clothes and "hit the treadmill—previously a place to store laundry," she says.

Receiving the diagnosis of Type 2 diabetes *is* a life-changing event. Adjusting to the news can take hours, days, months, or even longer. However long it takes is considered the normal amount of time.

2

SETTLING IN

Adjusting to life with Type 2 diabetes is a gradual process. It involves getting knowledge, altering attitudes, breaking old habits, and forming new ones. This sounds like a tall order, and it is, especially since medical advice can be confusing, even contradictory. Most experts agree that the key to controlling diabetes is a combination of diet and exercise, although some people with Type 2 diabetes also require oral medication, even insulin shots. Most experts advocate testing blood sugar levels, at least until you have learned how various foods affect you. (See chapter 3 and appendix 3 for more details on testing.) Unfortunately, there is little agreement on what makes up a healthy diet for someone with diabetes, or on when and how frequently blood sugar levels should be checked.

If you believe you're not getting the information

and support you need, you have plenty of company. This chapter will help you make sense of mixed messages you may receive from your health care professionals. You also will learn strategies for meeting the emotional challenge of true acceptance of your diagnosis and the life-altering changes you will have to make.

WHAT THE DOCTOR SAID

Some doctors write a prescription for diabetes medication immediately. Others suggest that their patients first try to control their blood sugar levels without chemical intervention. Some doctors treat diabetes as a serious but controllable illness—which it is—and see to it that their patients are counseled and trained in its management. Others seem to shrug it off with little or no apparent concern for the patient's ability to cope with the impact of having this disease, let alone manage it successfully.

When Vicki, forty-one, went to her doctor for a splint to relieve tendinitis in her wrist, she mentioned that she thought she had a urinary tract infection. The doctor tested a urine specimen, found a high level of sugar, and had the nurse do a finger stick (that is, draw blood from one of her fingers). A blood glucose test showed a reading of 235. "The doctor gave me a starter pack of pills and told me to take one tablet twice a day to control my blood sugar. But he didn't say whether I had diabetes or not. I was very scared and confused. I wanted to know if I had diabetes, but neither the doctor nor the nurse would answer me," Vicki recalls.

Each time Vicki went back to the doctor to deal with her tendinitis and urinary tract infection, the nurse checked her blood sugar, but the doctor wouldn't say whether the results were "good" or "bad" and never gave her a straight answer as to whether or not she had diabetes.

Vicki's doctor probably hedged about telling her she had diabetes to avoid upsetting her. For years she had been struggling with an eating disorder. Five feet, four inches tall, she had weighed as much as 325 pounds, much more than twice the optimal weight for someone her height, which is the definition for morbid obesity. Her doctor prescribed a drug designed to stimulate the release of insulin by the pancreas, and told her to take it twice a day to control her blood sugar, and said nothing about modifying her diet—perhaps because he thought that would be impossible for her. Since she also has chronic fatigue syndrome, he did not tell her the importance of exercise in managing diabetes, again no doubt assuming that her chronic fatigue or her weight would prevent her from exercising. Ideally, though, he should have given Vicki all the information she needed to develop a strategy for managing her condition.

Vicki's doctor may have thought that the very name of the drug—Diabeta—would suggest the presence of diabetes, but Vicki wanted a definitive, yes or no, diagnosis. Eventually, despairing of getting a straight answer, she insisted on a glucose tolerance test (see chapter 3 for details about this test) and finally got her diagnosis.

In contrast to Vicki's experience, Marcia's doctor told her right away that a blood glucose level of 181 meant diabetes, and that she should go on a low-carbohydrate diet immediately. Reluctantly, at Marcia's request, he prescribed a diabetes medication that prevents the liver from releasing stored sugar into the bloodstream. Like Vicki's doctor, he did not address the importance of exercise.

In addition to telling Delores to cut her food intake in half—advice that no one could reasonably be expected to follow—her doctor told her that exercise wouldn't help her. Delores knew better.

"It might not help much with weight loss, but I have read in plenty of places that it helps sensitize the cells to insulin," she says—correctly.

Mark was fifty when he got his diagnosis. His doctor gave him a prescription for diabetes medicine but no information on diet, exercise, or monitoring his blood sugar. Three years later, Mark came down with influenza, and, severely dehydrated, he went to the hospital emergency room. "When I told [the doctors] I was a Type 2 diabetic, they took my blood glucose. They couldn't read it on their meter. They sent a sample to the blood lab, and it came back at 1,171," he says. Mark was immediately admitted to the cardiac unit. He had been hiccuping constantly for five days. "They told me later that's a sign of heart attack in a diabetic," Mark explains. It took four days to rehydrate Mark. While in the hospital, he spent several hours with a dietician and was taught to use a blood glucose meter. By then, he says, "I had a new understanding and respect for what I was facing. And I got a new, competent doctor, too."

When Grant was diagnosed, his doctor gave him a prescription for an insulin-increasing drug, told him to make an appointment with the staff dietician, and informed him that "regular exercise was good." The doctor also advised Grant not to be so extreme about controlling sugary foods that he never allowed himself little treats on special occasions. Grant was to come in for an office visit after three months.

Greta was thirty years old and weighed about 350 pounds when she got her diabetes diagnosis. She quotes her doctor as saying, "You are diabetic. You must cut out all sugary foods immediately and take medication. You will probably have to go on insulin." But even though the doctor prescribed an oral medication instead of insulin, he still sent her for instruction on how to give herself insulin injections. "I was told to lose weight, but not how I was supposed to accomplish that, other than cutting out sweets and snacking," Greta recalls. Terrified at the thought of insulin shots, she took her pills and cut back on sweets "for the most part," but she resented being told to lose weight on diets that left her so hungry she couldn't stick to them.

"Over time, I got into a routine of taking my medication as prescribed," she reports. "I did eat some sweets, especially as time went by and it seemed that eating the sweets didn't raise my blood sugars any more than if I ate starches. I became complacent, but as long as I took my meds—in ever-increasing doses—my doctor said my sugar levels were 'acceptable.'" In 1999, after nine years of complacency—and benign neglect—Greta weighed 475 pounds. Most of the time she used a wheelchair. She had developed fibromyalgia, a condition involving chronic pain and nonrestorative sleep, and despaired of ever living a normal life. She sought the help of an endocrinologist, the specialist most often called upon to treat diabetes.

Gary, who read package labels in the grocery store in an effort to obey his doctor's instructions to "watch his sugars," continued feeling badly, so his doctor prescribed a drug that decreases the amount of glucose released by the liver. Three weeks later, still miserable and now plagued with nearly constant acid reflux (heartburn), he saw his doctor again. The heartburn made him almost totally unable to eat or drink. He had lost about fifty pounds in a few weeks and, although he didn't know it, was in a state of *diabetic ketoacidosis*, a life-threatening condition that can result from uncontrolled diabetes. "The doctor told me, 'You've got to give the pills time to work,'" Gary says. "Well, while I was waiting for the pills to work, I was almost dying." He was severely dehydrated. Finding a vein from which to draw blood was nearly impossible. When the nurse finally succeeded in getting a blood sample, his blood sugar level was too high to read on the doctor's office equipment. The doctor wrote a prescription for the heartburn and sent Gary home to wait for the lab results.

Driving home, Gary says, he felt as if he was under the influence of a drug like LSD. His head was spinning, and he could hardly focus his eyes. Later the doctor called and said, "We've got to get you to the hospital right away. I have to get you on insulin." It was the day after Gary's forty-seventh birthday. He was admitted to the hospital, where he lapsed into a diabetic coma for a short while. After he came out of the coma, the nurses at the hospital taught him to give himself insulin injections. He also met with a dietician and was shown how to use a glucose meter. "My life changed forever, but not in a bad way," Gary says now. "I got a great education at the hospital."

Of course, not all doctors are as casual about diabetes as Gary's former doctor was. Elaine had taken corticosteroids for five years to treat an autoimmune disease and watched with dismay as an uncontrollable appetite caused the weight to pile on. "I could eat a loaf of French bread between the store and home if there was a red light," she says. "My doctor knows me very well and knew that I could handle the news, so she had her assistant call me to tell me I had diabetes. The assistant gave me my test results, explained what they meant, and asked me to come in and pick up a packet of information. She suggested that I come on her lunch break so she would be available to give it to me personally and go over it with me. She also advised that she was making arrangements with my insurance company for a monitor and diabetes education classes," Elaine reports. "Since my numbers were not sky-high, the doctor wanted to see how much we could control [the disease] with diet and exercise alone, even though my exercise level is minimal some days. Once my monitor arrived, I was to test in the morning before breakfast, two hours after dinner, and at any other time I felt the least bit off."

Marissa's doctor talked mostly about potential complications of diabetes and referred her to a nearby hospital's diabetes education service, where she saw a dietician and a diabetes nurse-educator on several occasions.

Paul's doctor prescribed an insulin-stimulating diabetes drug and introduced him to the American Dietetic Association's food pyramid, which emphasizes complex carbohydrates and low fat intake. "What a joke," says Paul, the man whose fall off a motorcycle led to his diagnosis. "My problem is carbohydrates, so they want to put me on a diet that is 60 percent carbs." Paul decided to learn all he could on his own. He soon read that the drug he was taking stops working within five years for half of those who take it, "so I stopped taking it and switched to a low-carbohydrate diet," he says.

Rose also did her own research, after calling her doctor and learning he was on vacation. "I found the book *Dr. Bernstein's Diabetes Solution*, read it, and never looked back," she says.

THE ROAD TO ACCEPTANCE

In her book *On Death and Dying*, Swiss-born psychiatrist Dr. Elisabeth Kubler-Ross describes the coping strategies used by patients with terminal illnesses to come to terms with their impending death. Although diabetes is not a terminal illness, for many people the diagnosis is devastating and requires an extensive period of grief and adjustment. According to Kubler-Ross, there are five stages of grief: denial, anger or resentment, bargaining, depression, and finally acceptance. Not every person with diabetes goes through all the stages, and the progression is not necessarily in a straight line for those who do. People sometimes skip a stage and go back to it later, or bounce back and forth repeatedly from one stage to another before settling into acceptance and successful diabetes management.

DENIAL

The typical first reaction to the diagnosis of a chronic or life-threatening illness is denial, a shocked "No, not me." Dr. Kubler-Ross considers this reaction to be healthy, for it gives the patient time to regroup and develop other defenses and coping strategies.

For a week after her diagnosis, Alana blended anger and denial into a kind of temper tantrum. "I ate more sugar than I ever thought I could," she says. "It was like I refused to be diabetic. Just about all I ate was sugar." The huge carbohydrate intake soothed her emotionally but left her dehydrated and fatigued. Then she thought, "This is stupid. What am I doing to myself?" Realizing she was in denial, Alana decided to "just get back to real life." She started walking and exercising, and trying to watch her diet. She also took a class on diabetes management. "That class helped pull me back to reality," she says.

At first Carl simply refused to accept the doctor's diagnosis, despite the fact that at times he could barely stand up, and his vision had become so poor that he could hardly see things as close as sixteen feet away. Still, he says, "in the back of my mind, I knew that something needed to be done if I was to continue to live. In other words, I knew the doctor was right but needed some time to come to terms with the concept."

A year and a half after her diagnosis, Elaine is still stuck in denial. "I don't actually tell myself I'm not a diabetic," she says. "Instead I just kind of ignore it, pushing it to the back of my mind as I stuff that pizza down. And there have been times when I have bought things I shouldn't eat. I would tell myself it was OK, I have self-control now, and I can ration it out appropriately. That's a joke," she adds. "I can't."

Nearly three years after Marissa's diagnosis, she is still fighting denial, but her approach is to force herself to face facts. "This is my current battleground. I am taking many steps to keep the diabetes front and center in my awareness," she says. To keep herself focused, Marissa has developed the habit of testing her blood glucose before each meal and at bedtime and has incorporated her oral medications into her daily routine. She keeps track of her progress toward blood sugar management by calculating two-week blood sugar averages and recording them on a chart. She has met with diabetes educators and taken courses offered by a local health maintenance organization (HMO). She searches the Internet for reliable information sources. "For me, the solution to combating denial often lies in getting information and letting it 'stew' or 'ripen' within me. Then I come up with my own approaches," she says. Thinking about her relatives who have diabetes also helps Marissa combat denial. "I fear a heart attack, blindness, kidney failure, or loss of my feet—complications that have hit members of my extended family. I really want to avoid those problems, so I'm working hard to change my habits," she says.

For Barbara, who had no symptoms when she was diagnosed, denial for a while took the form of neglecting to use her glucose meter. "If I don't check my blood glucose, then there's no proof my levels are too high," she reasoned. "And if I feel the same as I did before I was diagnosed with diabetes, then I must not be doing all that badly."

For nearly five years Daniel did not work hard at getting his diabetes under control because he was in denial. "The process that brought me to my present state of awareness is this: My endocrinologist mildly chewed me out, pointing out that my current lifestyle was quite literally a form of suicide. Then my COBRA insurance—the health insurance employees are allowed to pay for when they leave a job—expired. While I was guaranteed 'portability,' because of my diagnosis I was placed in a risk pool that was very expensive and had very poor coverage, which jeopardized my opportunity to consult with the endocrinologist or other specialists. I attended a diabetes seminar that reminded me that my disease was either fatal or terribly debilitating if I didn't learn to control it. And finally, a close personal friend reminded me that these consequences were a matter of personal choice, within my control, and asked why in hell didn't I do something about it."

Vernon, who had the intermittent problem of the irregular heartbeat, heard his doctor's diagnosis but told himself he would be "normal" if he brought his weight down to a healthy level. "While my weight dropped from being on a low-calorie diet, my blood sugars did go down. So I started slipping back into my former eating habits and gaining back weight, which I also was in denial about," he recalls. He stopped checking his blood sugar levels, and his heart problem came back. "I ended up in the hospital with congestive heart failure and high blood sugars," he says. "The denial started to end then, but it took some more time for me to really accept that I would have to live with this in some form or another for the rest of my life."

Not everyone experiences denial, though. Rose, the nurse who diagnosed herself right after her mother's death, says, "Denial never once entered my mind. It's hard to deny a fresh grave—and harder still to deny the glucose readings."

Nor was denial an option for fifty-two-year-old Dee. An Alaskan aboriginal, she works for a native people's health service where many come to be treated for diabetes. "The disease can let you know if you're not taking care of it," she says, "and when you look at the effects diabetes has on your body, you know you have to take care of it or you won't be around long."

ANGER

When denial has served its purpose in giving the patient breathing room to gather strength, it's time to move on to the next stage: anger. "Why me?" the patient asks, and often, "Why not some other member of my family?" Patients may blame those who provide their health care, society at large, or even God. Selfish though it may be, this reaction is normal, even healthy, and should be accepted without judgment or criticism.

Anger can be a corrosive emotion, or it can spur you to combat diabetes's worst effects. "It's what keeps you fighting," says Roberta. "Anger is very helpful if you learn to use it to your advantage. And if some days you have a horrible 'brat attack' where you scream, and yell, and are so angry that you can and *do* spit, good for you. You are still alive and haven't given up. Yes, I am angry, and I use my anger. It's what makes me go out on a rainy day and walk two or three miles. I may not beat this disease, but I am going to fight back!"

People can find a variety of targets for their rage. Dee railed against her fate: "Why me? What did I do wrong?" Then she turned her anger outward. "I know I took it out on the people around me at times, not being able to control my anger, and just being mad all the time," she says.

Serena refused to believe her doctor for a while, but when she accepted her diagnosis, she recalls, she was "mad at the whole world for a time."

Carl's anger targeted the conditions under which he works as a social worker: "I was suffering burnout from the stress of my job: six or seven days a week, an average of fourteen hours a day; multiple daily meetings that were more like social gatherings, with coffee and cake; the need to be fairly sedentary, sitting at a desk. This replaced what was a reasonably active lifestyle, including regular gym visits, just a few years earlier. I think all of this contributed in a major way to the onset of diabetes. If it wasn't the total cause, it was at the very least a major factor."

Delores, who is disabled because of several health problems, had many targets for her anger but was surprised at what angered her. "I felt angry at my body for betraying me in yet another way. The diabetes diagnosis came a little over a month after a diagnosis of arthritis in my right knee, so I felt like I was getting it with both barrels," she says. "I felt angry at the chronic fatigue syndrome. It had caused me to gain so much weight, which contributed to the diabetes and arthritic knee. I felt angry at the doctor, who clearly had no idea how difficult losing weight is. I felt angry at having to do my own medical detective work and educate a doctor who should be educating me. And I felt angry at my health plan, which has no endocrinologist closer than a two-hour drive from where I live." The thing she expected to feel angry about but did not, Delores adds, was her heredity. Both her parents were Type 2 diabetics, but neither one developed the disease until after Delores was born. "I know they didn't deliberately choose to pass on those genes."

At first Barbara did blame her family, for making sweets the most desirable form of food: "My parents and grandparents gave me sweets to make me feel better whenever I had a boo-boo or was sad about something, as a means of distraction, and as a reward for being good. So I figured it must be their fault. They should have conditioned me to associate healthy foods, instead of sweets, with comfort."

Some blamed themselves. "I was angry with myself for getting into this position," says Gary. "I used to do everything to excess: drink, smoke, party all night. When you're younger, you don't worry about your health. Either you think you're going to live forever and you don't take care of yourself, or you get to a point where, when you're as big as I was, you think, well, if I die tomorrow, I die tomorrow—I'm going to live life to the fullest." While he was in the hospital, "hooked up to a bunch of tubes," he says he grew furious with himself. "I couldn't lay it on anyone else."

For a while, Mark did just that—blamed everyone but himself—before turning his anger inward: "First I blamed my wife's cooking, my kids' fund-raising candy bars, the tension at the office; in short, everything but the real problem, which was my stubbornness and refusal to face what my symptoms had been telling me."

For Rose, anger at the poor medical care that contributed to her mother's death was mixed with anger at her own situation. "I would be terribly angry about the medical misinformation that had my mom eating all the wrong things. I was angry that I got diabetes when I was only in my forties, and furious that my mother died when she was only sixty-three. I was upset that my daughter was alone with my mother—her grandmother—in a movie theater on her birthday when my mother died. I was angry about all of this all at once," she says.

Rightly or wrongly, many people reserve their purest anger for the very people they expect to help them the most—their physicians. Forty-five-year-old Walter, a network engineer, was angry at the casual way in which his doctor told him he was diabetic. "It was a sort of 'by the way' remark," he recalls. "She gave me no advice or instructions. I thought she'd just given me a death sentence. I didn't know a thing about diabetes."

After he was diagnosed, air force veteran Charles, the telecommunications analyst, realized he had been diabetic for years and blamed the military doctors for not recognizing this fact. Vernon did not become angry until he learned more about diabetes. "I realized that I was probably diabetic throughout the whole time I was having problems with heart rhythm and that my cardiologists never even considered a connection to high blood sugars. I did get angry then," he says.

Paul also had a delayed reaction: "For a while there was a certain amount of upset at the medical profession because I wasn't informed about the link between carbohydrates in general, not just sugar, and diabetes. If I had understood the role of carbs in raising blood sugars, I think I would have changed my diet a long time ago, and possibly even avoided Type 2."

Alana's shock at being diagnosed turned quickly to anger at never having been told that Native Americans have a propensity toward diabetes. (All she knew was that the disease ran in her family.) She thinks things might have gone differently for her if she had been given this information.

At the other end of the scale is Elaine, who says it never occurred to her to be angry: "I guess I didn't think anger would accomplish anything, and it uses a lot of energy to be angry. To some of us, energy is a precious commodity."

BARGAINING

Sooner or later, anger is replaced by a "Yes, me, but . . ." attitude. Patients try to strike a temporary truce, according to Kubler-Ross. This is an important step in accepting a certain loss of self-determination, while still trying to retain some control over the situation.

"The first thing I did was to try to bargain with the dietician, to get her to tell me just how much candy, cola, doughnuts, and sugar I could eat and not get any worse," Mark says. Alana, who received the news of her diabetes from her physician's assistant four days before Halloween, half jokingly tried to argue her out of it. "You tell me this on Tuesday when Halloween is on Friday. Halloween is the biggest candy holiday of the year," Alana said. The physician's assistant replied, "What do you want me to do, wait until after Christmas, and then after Valentine's Day?"

Alana got the point. But that didn't prevent her from making another bargain with herself. "I still do it from time to time," she says. "If I'm going on vacation for a few days, I'll tell myself I'll be reasonable, but I'm not going to be as strict on my diet as I usually am. Then, when I get back from vacation, I'll be really strict for a while, to make up for it."

Jill, who is forty and the custodian in an apartment house, took her diabetes diagnosis as a sign she was being punished and offered God a bargain, promising to "be a better person, go to church every Sunday, and be more understanding of others," she recalls. Barbara's bargain was to be "diligent about taking my oral medication," she says, "instead of giving up the foods I like."

Not everyone tries to bargain, however. Charles says, "I've been through this with God over other things, and I've learned not to play poker with

God." Roberta, who had seen so many complications of diabetes in family members as a child, states that bargaining never crossed her mind: "No other family member ever bargained their way out of this, and I was not even going to try."

GRIEF

Grief and depression are often the last stage before acceptance. According to Kubler-Ross, the person says, "Yes, me," having gathered the courage to admit what is happening. Sometimes termed *situational depression*, the depression that accompanies grief usually has a different quality from what psychotherapists call *clinical depression*. The symptoms may be similar—poor sleep, loss of appetite, difficulty in making decisions, and a sadness that seems never-ending. But even though both kinds of depression can feel as though you're enveloped in a dark cloud, the person with situational depression can usually identify its specific cause, whereas the person with clinical depression usually cannot. Talking about the cause, and the feelings associated with it, is good medicine for people suffering from grief and situational depression. Clinical depression is associated with a chemical imbalance and often requires medical treatment.

For Vicki, the sadness over her diagnosis accompanied a deep sense of loss. She had struggled for most of her life with compulsive overeating. After years of yo-yo dieting, losing weight and gaining back even more, Vicki had found a program called Overcoming Overeating (see chapter 5) and learned to control her food intake without feeling deprived or obsessive. So the diabetes diagnosis and its associated restrictions came as a particularly harsh blow. "I felt extremely sad that this happened. I feared that I would now have to give up all the foods I loved just after I'd made peace with them," she recalls.

Roberta felt a similar sadness. She remembers thinking, "A good part of who I am is gone." While she used to enjoy cooking, food had now become the enemy. Nevertheless, she needed food to stay alive, so it was a double-edged sword. Roberta was also sad because "it's hard to see your body betray you. While it can be helped, it can never be fixed and made whole again."

Helen went into an emotional tailspin when she got her diagnosis. Unlike most adult-onset diabetics, Helen is not insulin resistant. Her pancreas works, but the insulin it produces is insufficient. Because the doctor at first assumed she was insulin resistant instead of insulin deficient, gaining glucose control turned out to be more difficult than it would have been if he had correctly diagnosed the cause of her diabetes. "I'm a worrier generally, so I quickly became pretty anxious, even obsessive, about my diabetes. And I became quite depressed for a time when my sugars went off the rails a few months after diagnosis. At that point I started seeing a psychotherapist and went on an antianxiety medication for a few months. I'm more relaxed now than I was at first, but I think it would be fair to say I'm still fairly obsessive," she says.

A year and a half after her diagnosis, Helen is still grieving. She reports that she grieves "mainly for the loss of spontaneity this disease causes, but also for having to give up certain foods or eating such small quantities of them that it's not worth doing." She adds, "I also feel bad for my husband, for having to put up with my constant talking about my food or my sugar or my doctor's appointments, and for the loss of spontaneity in his life as well as mine because of my disease."

Rose was for a time overwhelmed with grief. "My mom was gone," she says. "She had lived with me, and I started every day reminding her to check her glucose level and take her pills. Now the equipment was mine and mine alone."

For many, the diabetes diagnosis came as a reminder of their own mortality. Rand, the writer, went through a bad time during which he doubted he would survive. "I thought I might be on my way out, and I started grieving over the things I hadn't done in my life. I had never really gone through the midlife crisis that a lot of people apparently go through. Suddenly, I realized there were a lot of things I really wanted to do—places I wanted to go, books I wanted to write. But now I thought I'd never live long enough to do them. Along with the grief there was a sense of fateful resignation."

Before his diagnosis, Daniel prided himself on his youthfulness. He had been the youngest member of his professional society and the youngest member of his state's legislature. "Being diagnosed with diabetes confirmed something I had suspected: I was getting older. This grieved and confused me," he recalls.

At fifty, Barbara found herself wondering how much more life she had left: "My husband and I were talking about retirement-related issues, and I found myself saying, 'If I live that long' and meaning it. I had also been thinking about how much time I would have with my grandchildren, when I eventually have some."

Marissa connected her grief over having diabetes with sorrow at nearing the age of fifty, changes in her menstrual cycle, and the fact that she never had children. "I grieved at giving up a long-held dream about how life would turn out," she says. "This is a feeling I reflect on nearly every day."

Margaret, a fifty-three-year-old photographer and artist whose day job is waiting tables, went through all the stages of grief and flirted with the thought of giving up entirely. "Believe me, the diagnosis was not an easy thing to swallow," she says. "I was devastated because I knew the restrictions I had to go through. There were days where, if I knew that my soul wouldn't go to hell, I would have given up and let my diabetes take over."

Walter says his grief was mixed with self-pity: "At first I was sad because I thought I had something like cancer. I was really feeling a lot of pity for myself. It wasn't until months after my diagnosis that I came to realize how treatable this disease is."

Elaine's grief was tinged with a fear of suffering from the same complications her mother had experienced. But she says, "My grief was short-lived. I learned that if I controlled my diabetes, I could avoid those complications."

Douglas, a forty-four-year-old tax consultant, also "grappled with grief" until he showed himself that he could make modifications in his diet and exercise to bring about an improvement in his health.

With a small dose of gallows humor, Norm keeps

his grief in perspective. He says, "I occasionally grieve for the pasta I can't eat, or for the chocolate cake or Ben and Jerry's ice cream I have to pass up, but that's the extent of grief. If I were to lose a leg, I might have some *real* grief to deal with."

ACCEPTANCE

Given enough time, most people facing death come to accept the prospect calmly, says Kubler-Ross. For those with a chronic but nonfatal illness such as diabetes, acceptance can mean the end of obsessive talking about it and the start of settling in for the long haul of management and discipline. The process of getting to acceptance may take a week, a month, a year, or longer, but eventually it will happen for most people.

Dee's acceptance of diabetes is typical. "I learned to accept it for what it is: a disease I will carry all my life," she says. "Just like a cancer patient who has been lucky enough to have the cancer removed, but is forever a cancer patient, you never get rid of diabetes, so you learn to live with it. It has become part of my everyday life, always there so that I must always be aware of what I do and how it may affect me."

For some, acceptance comes easily. Marcia, whose family history prepared her for the diagnosis, accepted the fact of her diabetes almost immediately. Similarly, Maria, whose Native American ancestry and two bouts of gestational diabetes served as a warning that she was predisposed to Type 2 diabetes, took the news calmly and began immediately to lose weight and stay free of medication. "When the weight came off, to my surprise, I was really happy," she says.

Elaine reports that she skipped all the stages of grief and went straight to acceptance. "It helped that it wasn't a surprise," she says. She remembers her diabetes educator asking how she felt about having the disease. "I told her that for me it was OK. It was just one more thing to learn to live with, and that I could do it." She adds, "I think that having other chronic illnesses made a difference in my ability to accept it, since my life has already undergone major change, and in comparison diabetes is a small one."

It took Walter about a week to accept his diagnosis. "I told myself there wasn't anything anyone could do about it, so I might as well accept the fact and get on with my life," he recalls. "After that it was much easier to look at all the information available, make a few life changes, and move on."

Sometimes a bad turn triggers acceptance. That's what happened to Barbara. After a series of good monthly blood test results at her doctor's office, she had one that was spectacularly bad.

"That's when I realized that this diabetes thing just isn't going to go away, and it obviously isn't going to control itself," she says.

Thad notes that he's about "seventy-five percent to acceptance" and quips, "I used to say, only partially in jest, that just because everyone in the past has died, that is no reason to believe that I will die also. I have accepted my mortality now."

Some people take an almost fatalistic approach. Paul says, "I can't change what is, so wasting my time and energy throwing stones at a brick wall is not going to do me any good." Similarly, Norm declares, "I made a quick mental calculation and said to myself, 'OK, this is it; now deal with it.'"

BEYOND ACCEPTANCE

After reaching a degree of acceptance, most diabetics begin to look more deeply into their relationship with the condition. Even those who felt most intensely that they had lost control of their lives and health start to look for signs that the situation isn't as bad as they had feared.

Often, progress does not follow a straight line. Marcia accepted her doctor's suggestion that she try a diet low in starches and sugars and high in proteins—the standard diabetic diet before the invention of synthetic insulin—and did well for a while. Gradually, she slipped back into her previous carbohydrate-rich diet, and her blood sugar levels slid upward into the mid-200s. Her vision became blurry again, and her energy level sagged. Spurred on by a few stern words from her doctor, she resumed her "low-carb way of life," and within two weeks her vision cleared and she actually began to look forward to her daily exercise routine. She now says, "I feel very positive and full of energy. I pray that I continue to have the state of mind that I do today—to keep going and not fall off the wagon."

Roberta continues to learn about the effects that various foods have on her blood sugar. "I still have a long way to go to figure it all out," she acknowledges. But she now knows that emotional swings and even minor illnesses can raise her glucose levels and has learned to roll with the punches. "I don't think you can ever have complete control," she says, instead of continuing to have temper tantrums in response to her disease.

Walter reports that he's getting used to the idea of being diabetic. "I don't like it," he says, "but I've learned to let people know of my needs, and they have been wonderful to me. I look at my situation and know it could be a lot worse."

Thad has set himself a goal: He wants to get his

blood sugar so well under control that he can get off medication entirely. Now he's taking one pill every third day and isn't sure he needs even that much. He will check with his doctor before stopping entirely but feels optimistic about his prospects.

One day at a time is the watchword for Daniel. "At this moment, I feel very optimistic, because I am engaged in a proactive approach involving strict diet, weight loss, and exercise," he says. But, he adds, "I've been here before and still have a foreshadowing of impending failure. I think my situation must be much like that of an alcoholic. Among other things, this means that if I think too far ahead, I will fall into self-fulfilling despair. So my goal is to maintain my regimen one more day, and my further goal is to renew this one-day vow tomorrow."

Learning that diabetes is a disease "that truly depends on behavior as one means of control" was a breakthrough for Elaine. "I settled down and started learning all I could about diabetes," she reports. "These days I really don't think too much about being a diabetic most of the time. I know I am one, and I live with that every day, but the difference is that at first I was so paranoid about everything that passed between my lips that eating became absolutely no fun. Now, while I would prefer not to be diabetic, at least it is something I have the power to control, and my eating habits are much more healthful than they ever have been."

Gary says, "I don't think of being diabetic every day now, but I know it's there, and I've changed my lifestyle to take care of it. There are very few diseases that you can say have made your life better, but diabetes has really changed my life for the better."

Rose admits that, to her, diabetes is still sometimes "a pain in the butt." But, she goes on, "I feel better, and that is wonderful. I have lost fifty pounds, and that is wonderful. I have knowledge and support, and that is wonderful. Does that make having diabetes wonderful? No. But still, it's OK."

Barbara sees her diabetes as an animal to be tamed: "I know that, through knowledge, eating style, preventive measures, and regular medical care, I can have a good deal of control over how I 'feed the beast.' I don't have to let it ravage my mind and body. I've put it on a leash and do my best to keep it there."

Control is the name of the game, too, for Teresa, a forty-two-year-old artist. Educating herself has been the key to her success. Says Teresa, "I control my diabetes. It doesn't control me."

3

LEARNING THE ROPES

Some people with diabetes want to know everything they can about the disease; others prefer to do what they're told to do and let it go at that. An article in the December 2001 issue of *Diabetes Forecast*, the magazine of the American Diabetes Association, describes how men and women differ in their reactions to having diabetes and tend to take different approaches to learning about their illness. Men are more likely to share some of the responsibility for diabetes care with their wives than women are with their husbands. Men are less likely than women to view diabetes as an illness, more likely to see it as one additional thing that needs to be dealt with as part of their daily routine. Women are more likely to focus on how diabetes restricts their diet and their life. Women tend to choose a treatment plan based on what is medically advisable, men on what best conceals their condition from associates. Whereas men are more likely to leave decisions about their medical care up to their doctor, women are more apt to question their doctor about the care instructions they are given.

The activist approach is fine for those with the time and resources—access to the Internet or a well-stocked and up-to-date library—to search out the information they need. The passive approach—following directions and learning only what is absolutely necessary—is fine, too, as long as your blood sugar levels stay within acceptable limits. What counts most is your mastery over your condition, not the way you have achieved it. Finding your own comfort level where diabetes knowledge is concerned is part of the process of gaining control over it.

Medical knowledge is not all there is to it, though. Developing the habits and routines that foster a healthy lifestyle is vital, but there are probably as many variations as there are people who have diabetes. This chapter looks at a cross section of learning and management techniques to help you develop your own, or refine those you're already using.

GETTING THE INFORMATION YOU NEED

Norm's attitude fits the male prototype described in *Diabetes Forecast*. "I generally don't pay attention to medical details," he says. "I heed what my doctor tells me to do, but don't listen to the reasons or the causes. I'm a great denier. The subject of illness bores me." It helps him, he adds, to take a mechanistic approach to his own body and get help fixing it. "I see my body as if it were a domestic hot-water system or a car. If something goes wrong, I call in a plumber or an auto mechanic—or a doctor."

Walter, too, believes the information he gets from his doctor is sufficient for him. "I just follow what the doctor tells me to do: take my pills and watch what I eat," he says. However, he hopes to be able to manage his diabetes without medicine someday.

Mark, whose blood glucose level at the time he was diagnosed was over 1,100, is more of an activist than most of the men surveyed for the *Diabetes Forecast* article. He decided his first task was to find a doctor he trusted enough to actually listen to. Then, he says, "I prepared for my office visits by writing down my questions. When she answered, I listened carefully."

Many diabetics rely heavily on the Internet to

get information about their disease. While Greg was in the hospital after his initial diagnosis, he saw an endocrinologist and a diabetes educator and got "lots of information." When he was on his own, however, he wanted to know more. "I had no choice," he says. "I felt I had to learn as much as I could. So I got on the Internet and found newsgroups and mailing lists. I got good information and support, and even found some friends."

Mark joined an Internet newsgroup to get answers to his questions from people like himself, only with a bit more experience at managing their diabetes. On-line, he read everything he could understand about the disease and the medicines used to treat it.

Appendix 1 presents lists of Internet resources dealing with diabetes, from electronic mailing lists to newsgroups to Web sites. When you come across other Internet resources for diabetics, heed this warning: There is no guarantee that the information provided is accurate.

Although Elaine used the Internet, she believes she profited the most from her sessions with a diabetes educator and a nutritionist. She had her first meeting with these professionals the day after her diagnosis. She also studied the information packet her doctor gave her, but says, "I still didn't feel like I had learned enough. So I went on the Internet and started reading and learning." She saw the diabetes educator and nutritionist three times each, arriving for her appointments with a written list of questions that often arose out of her Internet research. She recalls: "[They] patiently answered [my questions and] were probably the biggest help I could have had. They were there to help me and did everything to get me on the right track. The eating plan they gave me was easy to follow. . . . I have learned that if I mess up, to just get back on track at the next meal or snack time. But I think the most important thing I've learned is that I am in control."

Some people go to formal diabetes classes. Says Margaret, "Thank God for diabetic classes. Without them and my dietician, I wouldn't have made it." Alana had attended classes with her grandmother but found the experience was quite different when she was learning about her own case. "You miss a lot in a class when you're there as a caregiver rather than as the patient. So I learned a whole lot going through it a second time—and I'd probably learn even more if I went a third time."

Most hospitals and HMOs run diabetes classes from time to time. A phone call or two will probably be enough to help you hook up with one. Enrollment requirements and costs vary. Some classes are free, or nearly so, and open to the public. Others are for HMO members only or charge a fee to nonmembers. Some health insurance plans pay the cost, so it's a good idea to ask your doctor for a referral to a class he or she approves of. If insurance is involved, you can expect that the insurance company will want something in writing from your doctor authorizing your attendance.

Classes vary in format from formal lectures to informal question-and-answer sessions. However the class you attend is structured, you can expect an easy-to-understand explanation of the physical basis of diabetes, its complications, and how to reduce the likelihood that they will affect you. You will receive coaching in how and when to test your blood sugar levels and in keeping records. Depending on the audience for the class, you may learn about types of insulin and how to give yourself injections. You will surely hear about the available variety of diabetes oral medicines. Expect tips on exercise, planning meals, and other resources available in your community. But, since most classes are based on a curriculum provided by the American Diabetes Association, don't expect to be encouraged to follow any but that organization's high-carbohydrate food pyramid diet, which may be right for you, or may not. (For more details on diet, see the section "Eating Right.") Remember as you listen in class that knowledge about diabetes is continually changing. Exercise good common sense, retain what you find useful, and seriously question the rest.

Diabetes classes sponsored by Paul's health maintenance organization did not work for him because he didn't agree with their emphasis on pills and the food pyramid. So he decided to find out all he could about diabetes on his own. He recalls, "I searched the Net and bought books to try to better understand my options." When Paul began to direct his own treatment plan, his HMO doctor wasn't too happy about it; but now, three years later, the doctor accepts the fact that Paul keeps his blood glucose stable on a low-carbohydrate diet.

At first, Robert tried to follow his doctor's advice to "eat right and come back in a month for more testing." But after the first month, his fasting blood glucose level was still 350. At this point, he recalls, "the doctor scheduled me for a diabetes education class, put me on an oral medication, prescribed a blood glucose tester, and sent me on my way. The classes advocated the ADA food pyramid diet. I tried that along with the pills for about a month. But the result was a blood sugar roller-coaster that was difficult to live with." Robert started reading about diabetes on the Internet and found the solution that works for him: a diet low in carbohydrates.

Perhaps the most useful information for managing your diabetes on a daily basis is your blood sugar reading on a glucose monitor. Later in this chapter, we'll look at blood glucose tests as well as other tests commonly used on diabetics.

Gary, the motivational speaker at diabetes support groups, earns his living as an auditing supervisor for a grocery chain. He says controlling diabetes is like controlling a store's inventory. "I have auditors who work for me at retail chains—they count stocks, check the books, and come up with a figure to see if we are making or losing money in the store. I do seminars for managers on how to control inventories. And controlling inventories is a lot like controlling diabetes. There are certain things you do, certain practices that, if you follow these guidelines, you've got a pretty good chance of running a good inventory. Same thing with diabetes; if you figure out what procedures to follow, you're probably going to feel well."

EATING RIGHT

For the lucky few, the choice of what to eat and when is governed by their bodies' wisdom. These are the lean ones. They eat what they need, no more and no less. Almost all of us start life that way. As newborns, we cry when we are hungry, we stop nursing when we've had all we need, and we gurgle contentedly in our cribs until we go back to sleep, waking again when we need more nourishment. Studies have shown that small children, provided with a variety of healthful foods and allowed to choose for themselves without adult guidance, will select a well-balanced, healthful diet. With rare exceptions, we are born knowing intuitively the relationship between what we eat, how we feel, and how much energy we have.

But for many of us, that inborn knowledge becomes corrupted. Doting adults give us sweets and may teach us, without meaning to, to value them above other foods. We are invited to join in recreational eating: eating when we don't need to, eating foods because they taste good to us regardless of whether we need nourishment. Sometimes a person's working schedule or lifestyle dictates eating irregularly, on the run, or at odd times to fit in with the demands of the job. Until diabetes entered your life, eating was a simple matter: You felt like eating, picked whatever appealed to you or was most handy depending on your mood and how much time you had, and you ate it. Not everyone who behaves this way becomes diabetic—heredity has a great deal to do with it—but many do. Diabetes can turn you from a haphazard grabber of anything that comes to hand into a food fanatic.

If you talk with enough diabetics, the complaint you will hear most often has to do with planning meals. Some people, confronted with the fact that their food choices have got them into trouble, decide to eat as little as possible. "Eating became something I avoided," says Elaine. "I ate only because I had to, and not enough. I would take my food journal to the dietician, and she would just shake her head and ask me what I thought I was living on. But my blood glucose was great, and I lost ten pounds. It took her a while to convince me that eating was OK, as long as I made intelligent choices."

Making those choices is a chore Roberta would prefer to get rid of. "I hate having to plan out even the smallest detail of my meals now," she reports. "I can't just 'hurry up and eat.' I have to take a blood sugar test first, and see where I am, then, depending on my blood sugar reading, decide if I can still eat what I had planned on eating, or if I have to come up with a different menu."

People with diabetes have to be concerned about two consequences of dietary errors: having their blood sugar levels go too high or too low. The symptoms can be strikingly similar: Blurry vision, mental confusion, dizziness, and fatigue are the primary ones. People vary widely in what levels are too high and too low for them. For the average nondiabetic person, blood sugar levels between 80 and 120 are considered normal. But for someone with diabetes whose "normal" blood sugar level is around 140, a low of 90 may yield hypoglycemic (too low) symptoms.

Of course, oral medications play an important role in the blood sugar levels of those who take them. Some drugs are designed to increase the body's ability to use insulin manufactured by the pancreas. Since insulin's primary function is to store glucose in the body's cells for use as energy when needed, if you're taking a pill that increases the effectiveness of insulin and don't give your body food to make the glucose for the insulin to store, you are apt to "go low" and experience the symptoms of hypoglycemia. So eating on a regular schedule, keyed to when you take your oral medications, is crucial.

When blood sugar supplies drop too low, the liver can release glucose, stored in the form of glycogen, to bring sugar levels back up. But some medications are designed to prevent the liver from releasing glycogen to keep glucose levels from rising too high. Again, food intake has to be coordinated with medicine intake to keep things straight.

Travel, whether for business or pleasure, can make it difficult for diabetics to eat right. Grant's work requires him to travel and militates against anything resembling a regular eating schedule. "I can't afford to crash," he says, "so I err on the side of high blood glucose when I'm working. I snack. I have power bars and hard candy with me at all times. And I take sandwiches with me and eat them at my normal meal times, if I possibly can."

Like Grant, Gary has a job that puts him on the road a good part of the time. He visits the grocery stores in his chain, driving as many as 200 miles from one to another. "Preparation is the key [to diabetes management]," he says. "You've got to make sure you're carrying your little bag with your medicines and your [glucose] meter with you at all times." Before his diagnosis he would never take the time for a real breakfast before leaving for work. "I would eat on the fly," he recalls. Now he has breakfast at home before he leaves for work, and takes with him a cooler containing his lunch and some snacks, usually "a couple of pieces of fruit. I've got to make sure that I have a piece of fruit at around nine-thirty or ten in the morning," he says, "to bring my sugar level back up so I have enough energy."

If you're on the road and don't have good food with you, your choices are apt to be limited to what the nearest fast-food restaurant offers. Because it's hard to find healthy food there, Gary stresses the importance of making sure you have everything with you before you leave the house.

Eating in standard restaurants can be a problem, too, although as the prevalence of diabetes increases it should become less so. Some cooks add sugar even to vegetables, to make them more attractive to people accustomed to eating sweets. (The less sugar you eat, the sweeter many foods seem, and vice versa.) Robert, who takes no medicines and controls his diabetes strictly by diet, says, "I do have to be selective about what I eat, which makes eating out a challenge, but I've found that most restaurants let you substitute lower-carb items for starches. I usually say, 'Hold the potatoes, and instead give me an extra order of vegetables.' "

Alana, whose schedule causes her to eat often in the cafeteria of the hospital where she works, has learned to ask questions of those who serve the food: "I ask a lot of questions when I'm going through the line at a cafeteria. Much of the time the servers don't know the answers, so I ask them to go and ask the cook. I say, 'I'm diabetic, and I have to watch this. Please help me.'" Learning to do this wasn't easy for her. She explains, "At first I didn't want to call attention to myself and my diabetes. I felt they'd think I was whining or wanting special attention. Now, it's no big deal."

When Vernon first looked at the American Diabetes Association's list of recommended foods, he commented, "If I just eliminated the foods I like from my diet, what was left was what I could eat." Eventually, after two encounters with irregular heartbeat and congestive heart failure, he found himself reading about diets low in carbohydrates, an eating plan he had rejected for years. But this time, it made sense to him. "The restriction on high-carb foods was offset by the liberal amounts of high-protein and high-fat foods I could eat, and which I liked," he says. "I started on that plan of eating the day after my son's birthday party, when my blood sugar hit 350, and haven't looked back. Now I can tell people that I am diabetic without flinching or hedging." To be sure, Vernon would prefer to have no restrictions on what he eats. But he sees the crucial connection between diet and health: "Considering our unhealthy, high-carb way of eating in the United States, just about everyone will feel the effects on their body sooner or later.

I believe that I am lucky to have found out this way, rather than [having] a heart attack or stroke that could have been much more damaging."

Today, Vernon reports that his blood sugar levels are "very stable" and his heart rhythm is "very even." He no longer has food cravings and has lost forty-five pounds in a year's time.

One of the things about diabetes that makes it frustrating at first is that, regardless of what some of the experts say, there is no "one-size-fits-all" solution, no way of eating that works for everyone. Gary says that fats make his blood sugar spike, so he's gone from eating twenty-ounce steaks to measuring four ounces of uncooked meat, fish, or poultry, which lose about an ounce of water during cooking.

Some people need more time to find their way than others. Grace worked with a nutritionist for two years, searching for the right food combinations and timing of her meals, before she succeeded in bringing her diabetes under consistent control. It wasn't just what she ate that mattered, she learned, but what she ate at different times of the day. Like most dieticians who work with diabetics, Grace's nutritionist supports a diet high in complex carbohydrates. Grace controls her blood sugar levels by eating frequently. For example, in the morning she has breakfast at about

8:30 A.M., and a snack at 11, without which she is apt to experience symptoms of hypoglycemia. "My sugar level drops, and I get really shaky, so then I have to eat something to bring it back up," she says. When her blood sugar level gets too high, Grace uses exercise to bring it down. She says she maintains a high level of self-discipline for the sake of her adult children: "If they see me eating bread or something sweet, right away they worry, so I try to eat right for them."

Delores's technique for learning which foods affect her blood sugar has been frequent testing. "Getting the glucose meter and testing before and after meals was essential," she says. "I now know several favorite meals that I can eat with impunity, and with no need to test afterward anymore. I've learned that some carbohydrates must be greatly limited—white rice and popcorn, for example—and that I can eat others, such as blended brown and wild rice, yams, and refried beans, in larger portions. I have been eating significant amounts of protein with every meal for the last couple years, but I am still struggling with getting my meals on some sort of regular schedule. I get wrapped up in E-mail, and sometimes as many as seven hours can go by before I realize I need to eat."

Mara, a Hispanic woman who was diagnosed in

1998 and works part-time as a hairdresser, keeps a chart of the glycemic index on her refrigerator to help her make decisions about what to eat. This index measures the speed with which various foods turn into glucose in the bloodstream—that is, how quickly they raise blood sugar levels. Foods are ranked on a scale of 0 to 100 or above; the higher the glycemic index, the faster blood sugar levels will rise. The index was first proposed by Dr. David Jenkins, a professor of nutrition at the University of Toronto, Canada, in 1981, as a way to help diabetics determine which foods are likely to cause the least fluctuation in their blood sugar levels. Mara has done well eating most of her carbohydrates for breakfast—usually oatmeal and fruit—then working them off during the day with some rather vigorous exercise. A typical lunch for her is tuna salad with lettuce, tomato, and cucumber, and for dinner she will have meat and vegetables and sometimes beans or a tortilla. "I invest in myself," she says. "I buy the best food I can. I'm worth it."

Many factors contribute to how foods affect your blood sugar. Vicki reports she can drink a half glass of cola with a meal with little effect on a postmeal test, but the same drink between meals will cause a severe spike. "Ice cream is fine with me, but if I eat a hot dog, my blood sugar goes sky-high," she says. Even the way a food is prepared can make a huge difference: Some people can eat a potato baked but not mashed, carrots raw but not cooked, without a spike.

One of the lessons the glycemic index teaches is that the more processed a food is, the smaller the particles are that comprise it, and the faster it is absorbed into the bloodstream, hence the higher glucose spikes it causes. There are probably as many variations in what fits well and what doesn't with your goal of keeping your blood sugar level in check as there are people who have diabetes. The key, Vicki explains, is "to keep your control internal, to learn what your body can handle and what it can't."

People who can manage without oral medicines or insulin have an easier time with meal and schedule planning, since there is nothing besides what they eat to make their blood sugar levels go high or low. Robert says that now that he's hit on a diet that works for him, he no longer has to worry when he eats. In fact on weekends, he usually eats only two meals a day. But those meals are carefully chosen to demand little insulin and avoid the blood sugar spikes that come from eating sweets and starches, he points out.

Deciding how often to eat is an individual matter. Conventional wisdom in most Western societies is that people are supposed to eat three times a day. Alana reports that she does better eating smaller meals more often: “If I eat five or six small meals a day, I do better at controlling my sugars than if I eat three big meals and a couple of snacks.”

Douglas is blessed with a high tolerance for eating almost the same foods each day, something many people would find unbearably boring. Here is the low-carb diet that works for him: For breakfast he will eat almonds mixed in plain, unflavored yogurt with half a head of lettuce or a stalk of celery. Lunch consists of two small cans of tuna mixed with plain yogurt, and the other half head of lettuce or a stalk of celery. He describes the tuna mixture as “a tuna fish sandwich without the bread.” Dinner is a hamburger patty and green beans or broccoli and cheese, and an apple.

Gary, for whom a normal meal used to consist of a couple of plates of pasta, says the trick to managing diabetes is “to come up with a meal plan that’s not a chemistry class every night.” He measures his food: White foods—starches such as potatoes and rice—he puts in a one-cup measuring cup. Vegetables can be up to two full cups. A protein portion is three ounces of cooked meat, fish, or poultry.

When Raymond was a child, his physician father used to test the boy's blood glucose once a year, fearful that he would develop diabetes. He decided early on to learn for himself what to eat and what to avoid. He explains: "When my doctor said he wanted me to come back in three months, I realized that he sees four patients an hour, five hours a day. That's twenty people in a day, a hundred a week. In thirteen weeks, which is three months, he'll have seen thirteen hundred people. He's not going to remember me at all."

Initially Raymond relied on his glucose meter to tell him what to do. "I'd eat a low-carb meal and test my glucose in two or three hours. The next day I'd eat a plate of spaghetti and test my glucose every half hour. You've got to do that to learn what you can eat and what you can't. It's different for every person."

"There's no such thing as testing too much," Raymond declares. "You need to find out what foods are friendly and what foods aren't." For example, he says he can eat barley without a blood sugar spike, but not wheat. He's found a brown rice spaghetti that he can eat—"not every night, but every couple of weeks. I eat a little bit of spaghetti and a lot of meat sauce and cheese. It gives me a little spike, but not a huge one."

Raymond still takes oral medication, but changing his diet has stabilized his blood sugar levels enough for him to reduce his medication by one-third. “I’d like to eliminate my meds, but I don’t think it will happen,” he says, “and I’m not going to beat myself up if it doesn’t.”

In addition to constant testing to decide what foods he can safely eat, he has done a great deal of research on the Internet and by reading books, particularly with regard to nutritional supplements. What all this reading has taught him, he says, makes him believe in taking vitamin and mineral supplements. Also, he says that he finds a fiber supplement to be very helpful in controlling his blood sugar levels. “If I eat a meal that causes my blood sugars to spike and take a fiber supplement with it, I don’t get as much of a spike. Nutritionally,” Raymond says, “I treat myself very, very well. I don’t feel like I’m lacking anything.”

Occasionally, however, Raymond lets himself indulge in foods that a dedicated low-carb enthusiast would never eat—“a piece of sourdough toast, half a pancake, or maybe an eighth of a portion of potatoes,” he says. “It’s a treat for me, and I don’t shy away from it.” Giving up ice cream was a major battle in which he has declared a truce, not a victory. Despite his father’s near-phobia about diabetes, when Raymond was growing up, he, his sister, and their father had a bowl of ice cream almost every night at bedtime. "Now," he reports, "I'm down to having ice cream twice a month, and I'm fine with that. I'm better off to do that than to be battling cravings. And if I feel like having a candy bar, one bite is all I want. And that's all I'll eat."

TESTING

Doctors use a variety of tests, often in combination, to establish a diagnosis of Type 2 diabetes. One simple test is to dip a test strip into a urine sample. If the test strip turns color, it indicates the presence of sugar in the urine, suggesting diabetes. Most doctors consider this insufficient for a diagnosis and want to explore further. The next step may be a fasting blood sugar test, in which blood is drawn before breakfast. If the reading is higher than 125, some doctors will render the diagnosis immediately; many will want one or two additional fasting blood sugars before reaching a conclusion.

A fasting blood glucose between 115 and 125 is suspicious. The doctor may order an oral glucose tolerance test to obtain more information. This test is also done on an empty stomach. It involves drinking a solution containing either 50 or 100 grams of glucose. Blood is then drawn every half hour to an hour for two to five hours. People whose blood sugar shoots up rapidly and comes down slowly—an indication that insulin is not working effectively—will probably be told they have diabetes. Those whose blood sugar spikes and then drops suddenly—this may not happen until the third or fourth hour, which is why the test may last up to five hours—will probably be told they are at risk for diabetes. They may be instructed to monitor their blood sugar levels, just as though they had diabetes.

BLOOD GLUCOSE TEST

If the goal of diabetes management is to keep blood sugar levels within an acceptable range—and it is, although the range considered acceptable may vary from one individual to another—then the only way to see if you're achieving that goal is to test your blood with a blood glucose meter. And that means you have to give up a drop of blood to be tested, which entails puncturing your skin, which hurts. There's no getting around it: You have to test yourself—often at first, then tapering off (but probably never stopping entirely) as you learn how various foods affect your blood sugar.

Doctors and diabetes educators differ in the instructions they give their patients. Those who take insulin are usually told to test before each meal and use the result as a guide in determining how much insulin to inject before eating. Some health professionals tell their pill-controlled patients to do the same, even though they don't vary their pill intake depending on the results. Eventually, most patients figure out for themselves that they'll learn best if they test after they eat. Some test when they first wake in the morning, again an hour or two after each meal, and at bedtime or two hours after the evening meal.

Barbara, who takes an oral medication, tests her blood sugar four times a day. "Now, instead of what I eat determining my blood glucose levels, my glucose levels determine what I eat," she says. "I've learned some interesting things about my body by doing all this testing. For example, sometimes eating a peanut butter and fluff sandwich on diet bread affects my levels less than yogurt with fruit. Seeing how different foods affect my blood glucose makes it easier for me to choose my meals and snacks, which, in turn, gives me much more control and much more satisfaction than I had before."

Vicki, who requires insulin to manage her diabetes, tests her blood sugar four or five times a day—down from eight times when she was still learning the effects of various foods. "I test before each meal, then again two hours after I eat. And if that test is high, I may test again in another hour or two just to make sure my blood sugar is on its way back down. If it was still too high, I would take another shot of fast-acting insulin," she says.

Asked how she feels about sticking her finger so often, she said it doesn't bother her at all anymore. But it wasn't always that way. "The very first time, it took me about thirty minutes to do it. I sat there and just couldn't make myself punch the little button that activates the lancet. It scared me so badly," she recalls. "After a week or two you just start getting used to it. You learn which fingers hurt the most and that if you do it on the sides it doesn't hurt as much." Vicki has the process down to a science now. "My pinkies are out; they hurt too much if I stick them. I've learned that my thumbs don't hurt much at all, so if I have to do an extra stick during the day for whatever reason, I'll use my thumb." Also, she rotates the testing sites: "I've got my own little system where I use the outside of each finger on each hand and then I go back on the inside, so it's two or three days before I get to the same spot again."

Like Vicki, Delores was afraid of the pain of testing, but she found it "no biggie," she says.

Delores has a meter that draws blood from the forearm, where nerve endings are not nearly as prevalent as they are on the fingertips. She says testing with that meter is "pretty painless."

For Mark, a meter that can get blood from his forearm would be a great relief. Unlike Vicki, he can't switch hands to reduce the effect of repeated punctures. "I only use the fingers on my right hand," he says, "because I'm a musician and the fingers on my left hand are heavily callused from the steel strings on my mandolin." (See appendix 3 for more information on types of glucose monitors and selection criteria.)

Glucose monitors that can get blood from places other than the fingertips are relatively new. Some diabetes experts think they should be used at first in tandem with a more conventional finger-stick monitor, as a check on accuracy.

People who test daily sometimes see baffling fluctuations in their blood sugar levels: They haven't deviated from their dietary regimen, and yet their readings spike. There are several reasons why this can happen. Stress is one. The physical stress of a cold or infection raises blood sugar levels. Some people can spot an oncoming cold by a rise on their glucose meter. Studies have shown that excessive emotional strain lowers the body's response to insulin, leaving glucose in the bloodstream longer than it should stay. Daniel uses his blood glucose readings to remind himself of how he responds to "extraneous conditions, such as stress, business disappointment, or family disputes."

Sylvia, a retired registered nurse and an insulin-dependent diabetic, says that in many women the approach of a menstrual period causes blood glucose to increase. "I'd have to take more insulin for two or three days until I got past that, and then my blood sugar would go back to where it belonged and I would have to decrease the insulin," she says. Sylvia's late mother, also diabetic, lived in a retirement home. "At the change of seasons—spring to summer, fall to winter—her blood sugars would go out of control. I kept telling the nurses there, 'It's the change of seasons. You've got to up her insulin.' I was on the verge of going up there and giving her insulin secretly until I finally convinced them and they understood," she says.

Testing is how Alana discovered the effects that potatoes, bread, and other starchy foods have on her. "I test at different times to get an idea of how I react to what I eat. Sometimes I'll even test before and after a meal if I'm really having trouble. But most of the time I at least do my testing on a fasting basis in the morning." Alana's doctor told her to record the time of each test in relation to the time of her last meal. Because she works in a hospital emergency room, she can't always take her meals at the same time each day.

Raymond reports that he tests his blood sugars "as a formality" once each morning before breakfast. But twice a year he logs his food intake in detail and tests his sugar levels every half hour to an hour for an entire day, "just for the information." Once he conducted an experiment by eating the same breakfast as his future wife, except that he had much smaller portions of the starchy components, and then testing both his blood and hers an hour later. "I was up to 180," he says. "She was right at 100."

Gary says he no longer needs to test every day, as long as he maintains his regimen of measuring what he eats and exercising. By contrast, Norm uses testing as a motivator. He tests randomly before meals or at bedtime. "I deal with it as a daily competition between me and my blood sugar. I enjoy taking the test and monitoring the average. If I'm under 120, I win. I like to win," he says.

HEMOGLOBIN A1c TEST

Every diabetic should have a hemoglobin A1c test (HbA1c, or just A1c, for short) periodically. Your doctor should order the test for you every three to six months. It is especially important if you aren't testing your blood sugar levels regularly. It shows how well you've been controlling your diabetes over the past two to three months. Here's how it works: Hemoglobin (Hb) is a red-colored protein, the substance that gives the color to your red blood cells. It carries oxygen throughout your body. A small portion of the glucose that circulates in your bloodstream combines with this hemoglobin, in direct proportion to the amount of glucose in your blood. Once this binding occurs, a substance called A1c results. It remains until the individual red cells die, in two to three months. Analysis of your HbA1c gives an estimate of the amount of glucose in your blood and can tell you how successfully you are in controlling your serum glucose. The HbA1c result is expressed as a percentage.

A study of people without diabetes done in the mid-1990s showed that a normal, nondiabetic A1c is between 4 and 5 percent. Other studies have shown that diabetics who can keep their A1c at between 6 and 7 percent have a lower rate of complications than those with an A1c above 8 percent. A "good" A1c is worth striving for; your doctor can help you figure out what "good" is in your particular case. Says Teresa, "My doctor calls me her model diabetes patient. I was able to get my HbA1c readings below 5.5 within three months of taking strict control with my diet."

Not everyone can do that well that fast. Food intake is a major factor, but there is more to it than that. It took an A1c of 7.4 percent, after several in the range of 6 to 6.5 percent, to convince Barbara that her diabetes wasn't going to go away and she'd better get serious about controlling it. When Raymond was diagnosed, his A1c was 20 percent; four years later, it's consistently 5.6 percent.

THE R-TO-R INTERVAL STUDY

The vagus nerve, a name that's easy to remember because the vagus travels through the trunk of the body like a vagabond, can be damaged by sustained high blood sugar. This nerve performs some very important functions and can cause many problems, including digestive disorders and sexual dysfunction. Some diabetes doctors routinely test the functioning of the vagus nerve as part of an initial examination when diabetes has been diagnosed. The test, called the R-to-R interval study, is simple, quick, inexpensive, and noninvasive. It is performed much like an electrocardiogram (EKG), except that it uses fewer electrical leads. The R-to-R test, like the EKG, records the rate at which your heart beats. It draws a graph showing peaks and valleys, symbolizing your heart's activity. Each peak is called an R-point, and the distance between R-points indicates your heart rate. Normally—that is, if your vagus nerve is working properly—when you inhale, your heart rate increases, and when you exhale, it slows. If there is little variation between R-points on an R-to-R interval study, it is an indication that your vagus nerve is damaged. Some doctors order this study done at eighteen-month invervals to monitor neuropathy in this crucial nerve.

C-PEPTIDE TEST

One more test you should know about, although you may never need it done, is the test for C-peptide. C-peptide is a small protein, present in the blood, that is a by-product of insulin production. A person whose pancreas has quit producing insulin has no C-peptide. The test is normally used with Type 1 diabetics who are experiencing frequent episodes of hypoglycemia to make sure they are taking their insulin correctly. In theory, a person with an abnormally high level of C-peptide would probably be insulin resistant, since one of the effects of insulin resistance is for the pancreas to produce even more of the hormone. However, the usefulness of the C-peptide test in determining insulin resistance is still a matter of debate. Sylvia, who was first diagnosed as an insulin-resistant diabetic, used results of a C-peptide test to convince her doctor of what she already knew for sure—that she was, in fact, Type 1.

No matter how often you measure your blood glucose or monitor your A1c, it's important to keep in mind the significance of the resulting numbers: They're not meant to tell you how "good" or "bad" you are, how disciplined or undisciplined in your way of eating, or how long you can expect to live. Your test results are, however, an indicator of how susceptible you are likely to be to the complications of diabetes. Always remember: You're controlling your blood sugar to avoid diabetes's complications. Freedom from complications is the payoff for good control. Considering the potentially serious damage that high blood sugar can do to your vision, your circulatory system, heart, kidneys, and even your brain, monitoring and controlling your diabetes may come to seem a small price to pay.

EXERCISE

According to one of Newton's laws of physics, a body in motion stays in motion, and a body at rest stays at rest until acted upon by an external force. The "body at rest" part is certainly true for most people newly diagnosed with diabetes—and the external force is likely to be the diagnosis itself. There is no reason to doubt that the lack of exercise that characterizes most of us in this age of television and computers contributes to the upswing of diabetes throughout Western society. We drive to and from work, sit at desks all day, and sit some more in the evening watching television, reading and writing E-mail, or navigating around the Internet. Then we go to bed. Weekends aren't much different. Instead of sitting at our desks, we sit in easy chairs watching more TV or reading. We've come a long way from the days when our ancestors had to use their bodies to earn their livings.

Diet and exercise are crucial to diabetes management. Between 85 and 95 percent of all diabetics—depending on whose figures you believe—have Type 2, and the vast majority of them are insulin resistant. The best weapon against insulin resistance is exercise. Studies have shown that exercise increases the cells' sensitivity to insulin, reducing insulin resistance. What is not known is why this is so. As this book was being written, a research team at the University of Massachusetts in Amherst announced the beginning of a project designed to find out how exercise works on insulin resistance.

If your most vigorous exercise these days is climbing the stairs on the way to bed, hearing that exercise is essential to successful diabetes management must sound like a death sentence. You may have visions running through your head of lithe young things doing aerobics for hours on end. You may feel helpless and hopeless about ever exercising enough to make a difference. It's important that you know it's not like that at all. You can exercise enough to improve your health without becoming a major athlete. All it takes is the decision to get started.

The only way to get started is just that: Get started. How soon you will see an improvement in your blood sugar levels, and how great that improvement will be, depends on a variety of factors, such as how insulin resistant you are at the outset, how high your blood sugars are, how much you exercise, and how often you do it. There is no formula to tell you what to expect, but you may be pleasantly surprised to see your sugar levels heading south within a few days of beginning an exercise routine, and you're just about certain to see significant improvement within a month.

Walking is excellent exercise. The pace and timing are under your control, and you need no special equipment other than a comfortable pair of shoes. If you walk for five minutes, that's exercise. If you walk for five minutes four times a day, that's as good as walking for twenty minutes once a day. If you do that five or six days a week, give yourself a gold star—and watch your blood glucose meter readings improve.

If you live where the seasons change and poor weather conditions often make it difficult to walk outside, you need to do a bit more planning. Some people join health clubs; others buy a piece of exercise equipment to keep at home so they can't blame the weather for their inability to exercise. Some people simply walk briskly around the living room or climb up and down the stairs repeatedly. Listening to rhythmic music while you exercise, whether inside or out, is a good way to stave off boredom and keep up a good pace. Whatever type of exercise you choose, remember this: If you haven't been accustomed to exercising, start gently. Add to your routine when what you started with becomes easy (and it will). Keep in mind that even professional athletes don't increase their workouts by more than 20 percent at a time. You shouldn't increase by that much until you're in really good shape.

Greg is one of those who resists exercise, but he says he'll get started eventually: "I just have to get up off my hindquarters and get moving." Raymond isn't satisfied with the amount of exercise he gets—he walks a couple of miles a couple of times a week—but he's working on it. Mara, who lives where it's sunny most of the time, rides a bike three or four miles daily and has a treadmill to use when the weather is unfavorable. "The treadmill isn't as much fun as being in the street, though," she says. "I love riding my bike, with the wind in my hair and the chance to see all the beautiful flowers." On Tuesdays and Thursdays Grace goes to a pool and takes part in group water aerobics. The other days of the week she uses a treadmill, placed in front of her big-screen television set. She usually walks on the treadmill while watching a movie, so each exercise session lasts from one and a half to three hours.

For Carl, exercise is the major component in his diabetes management program. Getting started with a workout program was a major hurdle, though. "I didn't want to do it." he says. "Most days I still don't want to, but I now know that to seriously bring my sugar levels into check, I have to exercise. To keep them at acceptable levels, I have to exercise. To keep my HbA1c level at a point where the doctor won't have a heart attack, I have to exercise." It took a lot of exercise to get his blood sugar under control initially—"two hours at twenty-plus kilometers [about 12.5 miles] a day on the exercise bike, in two one-hour sessions." That level of exercise brought his fasting blood sugar levels to between 70 and 90. Now he can do just one hour and keep his sugar under control. He finds there is a residual effect that allows him to skip a day occasionally, "but on day two it starts to creep back up."

If you need motivation for exercise, consider this suggestion from Carl: "If you want to eat the occasional slice of chocolate cake, or if you're planning a meal high in carbohydrates, get on that exercise bike or treadmill or go for a jog beforehand. You should find that the resultant 'peak' won't be as high, which overall means better control." Note that Carl uses the word *occasional.* He's not saying, nor should you think, that you can use exercise on a regular basis as a substitute for good dietary control. The point is that exercise increases your body's sensitivity to insulin. If you're treating yourself to something that will require your pancreas to produce extra insulin to turn the treat into energy, extra exercise will help that insulin to do its work. But if you use exercise as a way to justify frequent indulgences, you'll fail at blood sugar control. You'll just become resistant to a higher level of insulin in your blood.

Even so, Grace is one who has found that exercise helps her deal with blood sugar spikes. She loves bread but eats it rarely because of its effect on her blood sugar. "If I eat bread, it really shoots it up," she says. "But then I'll go for a walk or get on my treadmill, and it brings it down right away."

Vernon worked his way gradually into a program of vigorous exercise. "I started walking, which gradually turned into jogging two miles a day, then three miles several days a week and two miles the other days, then to six miles on Saturday, plus less the other days. Then I added some weight lifting on the days I did two miles running," he says. "Recently I ran in a local 10K race and felt great!"

Daniel does thirty minutes of aerobics each day and some weight training. In all, he spends about an hour and a half each day in a gym near his office. It's a big investment of time, he acknowledges, but he thinks the results make it worthwhile.

Even if you've got your diet sufficiently under control that you don't need exercise to avoid blood sugar spikes, you can count on three other benefits from exercising. Although it may seem contradictory, exercise gives you more energy, not less. (That's because your cells are more sensitive to insulin when you exercise, and therefore they can accept more glucose, releasing it when you need additional energy.) Also, if you're looking to lose weight, exercise is essential. It burns calories and speeds your metabolism, the process of turning food into energy. Muscle burns more energy than fat, so building muscle through exercise helps you lose more weight more quickly. Finally, exercise leads to the release of endorphins in the brain. Endorphins are a group of proteins that perform two valuable functions: They are chemically the same as morphine, fit in the same nerve spaces, and relieve pain. They also help improve mood, so exercise is a way to help combat depression.

Gary knows all about the benefits of exercise. He avoided it for a long time, then decided to give it a try. "To lose weight, you've got to exercise—that's what everyone tells you," he says. "Well, call me stubborn. I played football in high school, and, even at 400 pounds, I could walk around the golf course, so I thought I was doing enough." But then he started running out of energy. "After a while, around the twelfth hole I started dragging. That's when I knew things were catching up with me," he recalls. At that point he says he was "still in the couch-potato stage."

When Gary had lost about 100 pounds, he started to wonder what it would be like to do a push-up without having his belly rub against the floor. "So I went down and did three push-ups," he recalls, "which was two and half more than I used to be able to do. I used to get down but couldn't get back up after that first one." Having succeeded at three push-ups, he decided to try to do a few more. Eventually, he worked up to ten push-ups. After doing ten push-ups a day for two weeks, he set fifteen as his goal. Today, about three years after he started, Gary does 125 push-ups in the morning, although not all at once. After seventy-five push-ups, he feeds the cat and starts his breakfast cooking, then does about fifty more.

At night, after work, Gary walks two miles in twenty-four minutes. That's five miles per hour. A normal, relaxed walking pace is about three miles per hour, which is fast enough for beginners. (Gary tried running, but it wasn't for him. "I just feel weird running. It's not in my nature to run," he says.) When he gets home from work too late to walk, he rides a stationary bike at a rate of three miles in ten minutes, "which is actually more of a workout than the walk," he reports.

Gary, who describes himself as a creature of habit, says, "[I do] something every day just so that I don't get out of the [exercise] habit. In the winter I like to cross-country ski at the local country club. It just feels great to be able to do it."

No one has all the answers to living with diabetes. Finding what works—what improves your health, what helps you to maintain an acceptable level of blood sugar and live a contented and productive life—is a never-ending process. If you view this process as a drag, that's what it will be. But if you tell yourself it's exciting to gain ever more knowledge and control over your health, you will come to believe those words and eventually to live by them.

4

JUMPING THE HURDLES

The road from struggle to success in managing Type 2 diabetes is dotted with hurdles and potholes. Your challenge is to get over the former and avoid the latter, while maintaining your physical and emotional balance. The good news is that you are not alone. Many people have gone before you on this road. While your solutions may not be identical to those you find here, in this chapter you will learn about the problems others have encountered, and how they are handling them.

STANDING UP FOR YOURSELF

Most doctors will encourage you and work with you so you can manage your diabetes to your satisfaction. But if you find that you and your doctor are at cross-purposes, it may be time for the two of you to part company. "Don't settle for second-rate medical care," says Barbara. "Not all general practitioners are able to provide the many facets of care, treatment, and support necessary for people with diabetes. Be loyal to yourself, not your doctor." She suggests seeing a diabetes specialist at least once while you are establishing your care regimen.

"Take charge of your disease," Greg urges. "You are the leader of your medical team." Sylvia, the R.N. diagnosed with Type 2 diabetes who finally proved to her doctor she was a Type 1, defines a diabetic's medical team as consisting of the person's primary care practitioner, an endocrinologist, a dietician, a podiatrist (foot doctor), and an ophthalmologist (eye doctor). She recommends that people who can't or won't perform daily foot inspections—including the soles of their feet—to look for injuries that neuropathy may keep them from feeling, should see a podiatrist every six weeks.

If you tend to be hypoglycemic when you wake in the morning, especially if you're taking insulin, your care team should also include someone who makes sure you wake up in the morning, advises Sylvia. Her husband leaves for work early, so a neighbor across the street watches their house to see that the curtains in the living room are open by 8 A.M. If not, the neighbor calls Sylvia. If Sylvia doesn't answer, the neighbor will call the emergency dispatch service, assuming she is too hypoglycemic to get out of bed.

Sylvia's training as an R.N. stood her in good stead by giving her the courage to challenge her doctor when he prescribed an oral medication that she knew might cause liver damage. The package insert recommended that a blood test for liver function should be done before starting the medication, and every two months for the first year.

So Sylvia wrote a letter to her doctor, enclosing a photocopy of the package insert and asking for a liver function test before starting the medicine. The doctor called her and said he didn't think the test was necessary, pointing out that she'd had one a few years before and it was normal. Sylvia recalls the rest of their conversation: "'Well,' I said, 'I'm not going to take it unless we do a liver function test. How do you know I'm not a closet alcoholic and my liver is shot?' He was very condescending, but he gave me the referral. He's a good doctor," she adds, "but he's having a hard time dealing with a person who has educated herself and maybe knows a little more than he does about diabetes."

Delores is another person who took the time necessary to educate herself about the various oral diabetic medicines, their mechanisms, and their possible side effects. "Since I used to be hypoglycemic and I have a high fasting insulin, I wanted to be sure I was not given a medicine that stimulated production of more insulin or caused frequent hypoglycemic incidents," she explains. The doctor she saw to get her prescription dug some samples of an oral medicine out of his pocket and gave them to her. "When I questioned him about its effect on insulin and hypoglycemia, he said he hadn't heard of any problems. I looked it up on the Internet as soon as I got home, and sure enough, it was exactly the wrong medicine for me."

She called the doctor's office immediately and talked with the nurse, who said Delores must have looked the drug up on the Internet, because they didn't have any information on it. Delores remembers asking, "What is the doctor doing giving out medicines for which he has no information?" The doctor then came on the phone and told Delores to research the medicine that would be best for her. She said she already had and named a first and second choice as possibilities. She drove back to the doctor's office and swapped the samples he had given her for samples of her first choice, which is making a decided improvement in her condition. "I've learned from the Internet list I'm on that this kind of experience isn't unusual," she says.

Greta stresses balancing your doctor's advice against what you know about yourself and what you can learn on your own. "Don't blindly accept whatever your family doctor tells you," she says. "See a specialist, at least for an initial consultation and workup." She says people who belong to HMOs or other managed-care plans are often told they don't need to see a specialist because the primary care doctor treats plenty of diabetics. "That may be true," she says, "but they are not specialists. Take your health into your own hands, get advice from an endocrinologist or other diabetes specialist, and educate yourself."

Teresa says, "My personal take on a lot of doctors is they are ill informed about diabetes. They seem to want to push medicine to 'solve' the problem. . . . I've been lucky that my doctor trusts me to make the decisions for my best health. She is very supportive because my blood glucose levels prove what I'm doing is working—and who can argue with success?"

Gary shares his number one rule about doctors: If your doctor says you are diabetic but doesn't send you to meet with a nutritionist and tell you to get yourself a blood glucose monitor, run as fast as you can away from that doctor. Without the monitor and nutrition information, you're lost." And for Marissa, the key is to "stay close with your doctor. If you don't have one you can talk to and who respects you, search for another. Be an active member of your health care team—in fact, be the leading member."

OBSTACLES TO EXERCISING AND LOSING WEIGHT

In addition to diabetes, Delores has chronic fatigue syndrome, an ailment that saps her energy. She wants to exercise, both to improve her cells' sensitivity to insulin and to help her lose weight, but like most people with chronic fatigue syndrome (and unlike most others), she feels worse after exercise than before. "Serious exercise is out of the question," she says, "although I do have a morning 'rocking chair workout' I do almost every day." Doctors recognize rocking as good exercise. Former president John F. Kennedy, who suffered with low back pain and other musculoskeletal problems, kept a rocking chair in the Oval Office at the suggestion of his personal physician. Delores says she started by rocking for twenty minutes at a slow pace, keeping time to slow, relaxing music. She gradually increased the length of each workout as well as her speed, then added a set of arm lifts, neck stretches, and torso twists that she does as she rocks. (See appendix 4 for in-home and seated exercise videotapes.)

Because people with chronic fatigue syndrome often tolerate water exercise better than other forms, Delores plans to expand her workout to include exercise in a water therapy pool. Many YMCAs set aside pool time for people too out-of-condition to do much exercise, but it doesn't take an exercise therapist to get you moving. Just find a pool where you can walk back and forth in chest-deep water, swinging your arms naturally, against the water's resistance. You can do gentle stretches, range-of-motion exercises, and leg lifts, standing at the side of the pool and holding on to the ledge or steps for stability. You can also use Styrofoam dumbbells or a foam kickboard to push against the water's resistance. A range-of-motion class for people with arthritis may help you kick-start your exercise program. The key is to start gently and work up gradually to a more demanding exercise routine. You'll be surprised at how soon you see an improvement in your energy level, a sign that your cells are making better use of the food you eat, which means your insulin resistance is decreasing.

Like many people, diabetics and nondiabetics alike, Marissa finds the greatest obstacle to exercising is making it an integral part of her daily routine. “I have to get more structured about my life,” she says. “It’s like a leopard changing his spots. Or, more precisely, teaching an old dog new tricks. Truthfully, I wish I didn’t have to [exercise]. But I fear a heart attack, blindness, kidney failure, or loss of my feet—complications that have hurt members of my extended family. I really want to avoid those problems, so I am trying to change myself and my habits.”

Often, the obstacle to weight loss is an imbalance between diet (calories taken in to fuel the body) and exercise (calories burned through physical activity). For weight loss to occur, there must be a deficit in calories—that is, more calories burned than ingested. Daniel struggles with this obstacle. A bit over five feet ten inches tall, he has weighed 260 pounds for the past ten or fifteen years and can’t seem to lose weight, although he knows he should. He’s trying to increase his exercise and decrease what he eats. “The diabetes consultants I’ve talked to say I can get rid of the weight, and the endocrinologist says it’s not going to be easy to get rid of but I will if I stick with my program, so I’m hopeful,” he says.

Finding “genuine support” from others facing

the same issues can take a while. Barbara's experience with support groups was disappointing. "Most of them are nothing more than petty competitions," she says. "The one who loses the most weight by the next meeting gets a pretty little pin that does little more than say, 'I succeeded, and you failed.'" To meet her needs for sociability and support, she joined several on-line groups dedicated to dealing with diabetes and healthy lifestyles. She says, "It's amazing how honest, sincere, and helpful people are when there are no contests for them to lose and when they can maintain some level of anonymity."

The problem of compulsive overeating is such an important topic that an entire chapter is devoted to it. If compulsive overeating is keeping you from losing weight, be sure to read chapter 7.

LEARNING TO EAT AGAIN

Eating is something we have to do to stay alive, but it's much more than that. Almost any time people get together, food is apt to be present. In every culture eating is a social act, a way of acknowledging your humanity and the humanity of those with whom you share food. We eat together to celebrate happy occasions and to console ourselves when we mourn. We show others that we honor their ethnic heritage by eating their special foods. We eat when we're hungry and, to be polite, when we're not. Recreational eating is as much a part of Western culture as football, hockey, or going to the movies. And that presents a problem. For many people with diabetes, recreational eating, eating to be sociable, has played a large part in causing their illness.

For the first couple of months after her diagnosis, Elaine gave up eating out, something she had done with her friends nearly every Monday evening for years. Still learning to control her food intake, she was afraid she'd "overindulge" and lose the discipline she was trying to develop. When she learned that her HbA1c had dropped two points in two months, she realized she was doing well. Her doctor reminded her that it was all right to eat out, and that if she occasionally strayed from perfection, she could mend her ways the next time she ate.

"I've always been such a good chow hound. I would say yes to nearly anything anyone offered me—and it shows," Elaine says. "Once I was diagnosed with diabetes, I had to start saying no, which originally met with resistance—both from me and my host. But I did it, and after a while saying no became a habit, and now whatever is being offered—usually a rich dessert—doesn't even make me drool most of the time."

Elaine also has learned how to control the amount of food she eats. When she shops for groceries, she says, "I've learned to read labels carefully. I've come to realize that what is listed as a portion on the nutrition facts label may well be twice what I want to include in my meal." During the two months when she gave up eating out with her friends, she measured everything she ate. Now, every few months—or more often if her blood sugar level starts "creeping up"—she checks portion sizes again by measuring everything for a week or so.

And when she eats out, Elaine uses her experience measuring portions to estimate the size of the portion on her plate. She thinks about the ingredients likely to be in the dish she orders, and takes them into account in estimating her intake. "I've also finally learned that leaving food on my plate is OK," she says, "or that I can take some of it home if it's something I would enjoy as a leftover."

For the friends who still "don't get it, when they offer me desserts, fries, pasta—things that aren't as good for me as they should be—I ask them, 'How many carbohydrates per serving?' and if they don't know, I only take about a tablespoon and fill up on salad or vegetables." Elaine is still eating with her friends, still being sociable, only now she's taking care of herself while she does so.

For Barbara, the big realization that came along with her diagnosis was how little she understood the specifics of diabetes—particularly the relationship between food intake and blood sugar levels. She has come to welcome the ongoing learning process. Her primary information source is the Internet, but she has learned to be cautious about the reliability of information she finds there. She says, "I will continue to use reputable Internet sites to gain knowledge at my leisure, in the comfort of my home." Barbara worked with a registered dietician to analyze her eating style and determine what further adjustments she needed to make, and decided to make those changes gradually, so she wouldn't feel as if she was punishing herself.

Some obstacles remain for Barbara. "I need to think before I eat; to make sure I don't run out of medication, lancets, or test strips; to remember to take my glucose monitoring kit everywhere I go; to take extra safety precautions because of my body's decreased ability to fight infection and disease; and to make sure I can eat within certain time frames. For some reason," she explains, "if I don't start eating my evening meal by six, my postmeal blood glucose will be higher than if I had eaten the same meal a little earlier." Barbara accepts that there is no scientific explanation for this, while continuing to hope that someday there will be.

Many people with diabetes say their biggest problems relate to cravings for favorite foods. Charles, whose blood sugar levels have gone from 350 down to 120, says overcoming his chocolate craving was a big factor in his fight to control diabetes. "There are plenty of diabetic chocolate bars and shakes," he says, and "plenty of other good things out there that are low in sugars and carbs."

Delores overcame her craving for sweets that she knows she can't handle—ice cream, for example—by including more protein foods in her meals and being creative with low-carb baking and cooking. She also makes a point of having favorite foods prepared and on hand, to help her avoid the foods she shouldn't be eating. "It particularly helped me to identify what characteristics of the 'forbidden' food turned me on, so I could find an appropriate substitute," she says. "Triscuits with unsweetened peanut butter get me through a yearning for cookies, because they're crunchy and rich. A thick chocolate protein shake, with some Neufchâtel cheese and ice cubes, takes care of ice cream cravings."

Rose shuns chocolate ice cream, her favorite flavor, by convincing herself it looks unattractive.

Barbara has adopted the strategy of trying to make the meals she sets before her family appropriate for her diabetes and their tastes at the same time. "I've dedicated some of my kitchen space for the display of a seemingly never-ending assortment of herbs and spices—about forty so far—and will add new items as I find them. I hunt on the Internet and in cookbooks for recipes worth adjusting to a diabetic's needs. And I'm trying to get my family more actively involved in the recipe research and actual cooking process."

DEALING WITH COMPLICATIONS

Diabetic neuropathy and poor blood circulation are very common problems among people with diabetes. Neuropathy occurs most commonly in the feet, causing dry skin, numbness, and tingling, and contributing to the danger that a foot injury will go unnoticed and cause infection. Elevated blood sugar levels can impair the working capability of nerves; the process happens slowly and appears to be reversible, at least some of the time. High blood sugar also damages blood vessels, especially the tiny capillaries that bring oxygen and nourishment to the eyes, kidneys, and feet. Diabetic dementia, which seems much like Alzheimer's disease, can result from long-standing unregulated blood sugar and the damage caused to nerves and blood vessels in the brain. Sexual dysfunction stems from damage to nerves and blood vessels in the genital area. (See chapter 6.)

GASTROPARESIS

People who live with undiagnosed diabetes for years can develop neuropathy in the vagus nerve, which controls the emptying of the stomach after a meal. Vagus nerve neuropathy results in gastroparesis, or delayed stomach emptying. It may cause no symptoms at all, or it may result in unpleasant symptoms after meals, including heartburn; pain in the abdomen, stomach, or chest; belching, bloating, nausea, and vomiting; constipation, sometimes alternating with diarrhea; a feeling of fullness after eating only part of a meal; and hypoglycemic symptoms such as fatigue and mental confusion.

Gastroparesis may not happen after every meal, but a person who has any other form of diabetic neuropathy probably also has delayed stomach emptying at least some of the time. Rand has this problem, but he's on the way to solving it. "Last year," he says, "I was getting intense pain in the stomach and a sense of weight or pressure around my esophagus. Sometimes the pain would hit me hard, and if I was driving I'd have to pull over to the side of the road." Rand's father had died at fifty-four of complications resulting from an ulcer, so the thought of stomach problems was particularly distressing to Rand. His doctor ordered extensive tests of just about every abdominal organ, with no definitive results. "The doctor was ready to throw up his hands. He couldn't come up with a clear-cut reason for the pain," Rand says. Finally, the doctor decided to try a stomach-emptying test and hit the jackpot. Rand's vagus nerve, which controls the opening of the pyloric valve between the stomach and the small intestine, had developed neuropathy. Sometimes Rand's stomach would empty its contents promptly, as it should, but most of the time it didn't, and pain resulted. "Instead of my stomach taking half an hour to empty, it was taking hours," Rand says. His doctor said nothing could be done but suggested Rand eat smaller meals more often during the day and avoid red meat and alcohol because they were adversely affecting his digestive process.

Even if there are no symptoms, gastroparesis can cause problems with blood sugar control, especially if you are taking medication or injecting insulin. Most drugs are timed to be most effective when the stomach empties its contents into the small intestine, from which nutrients and glucose are absorbed into the bloodstream. "The problem the gastroparesis causes is that it holds the food in your stomach and doesn't release it gradually," Rand explains. "Instead, it may dump it into your gut all at once an hour or two after you've eaten. So then the question is whether the medication you took with your meal will still be working when the glucose hits your bloodstream." If an agent designed to lower your blood sugar hits your bloodstream when your blood sugar isn't elevated from having recently eaten, the likely result is a hypoglycemic episode, which can involve shaking, cold sweats, and—worst of all—sleepiness. It's quite likely that many people who fall asleep at the wheel while driving are experiencing hypoglycemia.

Gastroparesis can also have an impact on when and how you exercise. It's not comfortable to exercise when your stomach is full, and with gastroparesis that condition can last for hours. Adding exercise when you are already hypoglycemic can cause unpleasant reactions such as headache, dizziness, and fainting.

Rand, whose doctor didn't order an R-to-R interval study (see the "Testing" section in chapter

3), tried the doctor's suggestions to eat small meals and limit red meat, to no avail. One day, in a bookstore, he came across a book that had a chapter on gastroparesis. The book recommended a reduced carbohydrate diet, and when Rand cut back on his intake of starches and sugars, he says, "it took about two or three weeks, and things started to improve and improve, and it just kept going. Suddenly, I felt like I could walk around again, and that's when I started to get more active and do more exercise." The key to defeating gastroparesis, as well as other types of neuropathy, is to keep your blood sugar within normal range all the time, and that means avoiding those foods that cause spikes.

FOOT PROBLEMS

People with diabetes are more prone to infection, and an untreated foot injury that becomes infected can require surgery and put you out of commission for weeks. In the worst case, amputation can be required. There's no reason to let this happen when simple precautions can prevent it. Some communities have free or low-cost foot clinics on a regular basis where people can have their feet inspected by a professional and their toenails trimmed, avoiding one of the most common causes of foot injury in diabetics. A call to your local Council on Aging will help you find out if such a clinic is held near you.

DEPRESSION

As we saw in chapter 2, situational depression is a normal part of the grief stage that must be worked through before coming to terms with the fact that you've been diagnosed with diabetes. Yet depression is often a by-product of diabetes itself. It sometimes starts before the diagnosis and more often occurs in the first few years after the diagnosis. (See page 45 for common symptoms of depression.) It's hard to stay motivated to care for yourself when you're depressed, but your very life may depend on it.

The key to solving this problem may be to force yourself to act *as if* you are motivated, even though you are not. If you make a list of things you would do if you were motivated to manage your diabetes, you may be able to use that list as a prompt on your worst days to see you through them without getting out of control. Writing things down—your thoughts and feelings and especially how they are related to what you eat—is an excellent technique for gaining control over your emotions and what you eat. You may find that you're eating out of rebellion, or to comfort yourself when you don't really need to, or because you're bored and want to stimulate your senses. You may put your finger on a problem that, in reality, you can work toward solving, and once you do, your depression may lift.

Don't forget that exercise is a way to fight depression. As noted in chapter 3, the endorphins released in the brain during exercise help improve your mood. Depressed people often turn to carbohydrates for comfort, which may help for an hour or two but is self-defeating in the long run because of the negative effect extra sugars and starches have on weight and blood sugar levels. Similarly, alcohol, a carbohydrate, may numb the pain of depression for a while, but its real effect is as a depressant. Be sure to see the discussion of insulin and serotonin levels in chapter 5.

When, despite your best efforts, you can't beat depression on your own, it's a good idea to go for counseling (to relieve situational depression) or see a general physician or psychiatrist (who can prescribe medication to correct the chemical imbalance associated with clinical depression).

INTERPERSONAL RELATIONSHIPS

The people with whom you spend your time at home, in social settings, and at work can be your best assets or worst liabilities when it comes to living with diabetes. They can support—or sabotage—your efforts at control. It's usually in your best interest to assume that people who are unhelpful are acting out of a well-meaning but misguided effort to be helpful. With that attitude, you can show them in a clear but nonchallenging way how their words and actions affect you. Then, if they don't change their ways, you will have to decide how much you want to let them into the part of your life that involves diabetes. If you're having trouble with people who don't understand what you're dealing with, remind yourself that others have dealt with the same problems. Try not to get discouraged while you work on them yourself. Ultimately, you have to take responsibility for your own diabetes, but it helps if those around you cooperate, so it's in your best interest to teach them what you need and how they can help you.

It's not easy to explain to people how diabetes works, and how it affects almost every aspect of your life. It is an invisible illness. You don't look sick. Barring extremes, you don't look any different when your blood glucose is too high or too low. You may know that you can eat certain foods at some times but not others. And if you do, you'll know when those times are, but nobody else can possibly guess. The lack of rigidity about eating that can make diabetes more tolerable can also baffle those around you, making them feel frustrated and guilty about not fully understanding your needs. They may not understand—how could they?—why you can go out for pizza one night and not another.

Barbara's husband used to show his affection by bringing home candy bars for the two of them to share. "His intentions were good, but I finally had to ask him to stop," she says. "Now I think it confuses him that sometimes I can have one but other times I can't. He buys them for himself but thinks he has to hide them from me. I think he feels guilty about having them around me. I tell him it's OK, but he still feels guilty eating them when I can't." Sometimes, too, her friends at work will bring her a favorite pastry or doughnut "as a gesture of kindness. They are registered nurses and know I have diabetes, but, because I eat so many of the same foods they do, they sometimes forget about it. There are times I can eat what they bring, and times I can't. When I can't, I make a sort of joke of it by saying something like, 'What are you trying to do, kill me? That's it. I'm taking you out of my will.'" Laughing, Barbara will then thank them for their kindness and say she's not hungry but will save the treat for later. "They apologize, and I tell them not to worry about it because now I have something to look forward to in the evening. I take it home, and sometimes I'll eat it, other times I won't."

Diabetes is a family affair where Rose is concerned. Her daughter learned to recognize numbers by reading Rose's glucose meter. Her teenage son calls the meter "the alien contactor." "We make jokes about it," she says, "but we all know it is a serious matter. Even my seven-year-old daughter knows what a 'bad' number is. I had to explain to her first-grade teacher why my daughter didn't want to be the number 200 in an exercise in counting. Around here, 200 is a bad number."

Some people find family members the hardest of all to deal with, but that's not always because of things they say or do. Marcia says her trouble with her family is at least in part because of her own attitude. "I have a problem sharing this diagnosis with my family," she explains. "I feel I should have known better, since my mom died from complications of diabetes. I don't want them to feel that I will continue down the same path as my mom, and I don't want them to worry about me." Yet many of her relatives, as well as friends and work associates, fail to understand her dietary constraints. "They all seem to think 'just a little' is OK for me," she complains.

Roberta can come up with a whole list of comments that well-meaning people have made in response to her diabetes. Here are a few examples: "My uncle couldn't eat peas. Maybe you should give them up." "My cousin can't eat carrots. Have you thought about that?" "You have to stop eating that. It's bad for you. You're doing it all wrong." "My doctor has me on a better medication. If I were you, I'd get a different doctor."

"It never stops amazing me that we can have the same disease, but with each person, the fine-tuning is so very different," Roberta says. "You have to learn to let [these comments] go in one ear and out the other. If you don't, these well-meaning people will drive you crazy."

Walter, who says for the most part the people who surround him have been "wonderful," admits to problems with meals at home. "I can't get my family to support a healthy diet. We eat really poorly because of my wife and fourteen-year-old son," he says. Asked what he does about this problem, he says, "Nothing. I just have to work around them." He's found great support, he says, from friends, "especially the ones who now tell me they are diabetic and I didn't know."

Since diabetes runs in Margaret's family and her relatives are aware of the problems it presents, she doesn't have to teach them about the disease. And when she got her diagnosis, her companion made it his business to educate himself. At work, she says, "it's a different story. Most people are indifferent to the situation, although some are sensitive to my problem. Most see my diabetes as just another disease."

Mara feels pressure in social situations with her family and friends. "My sister-in-law gets after me. She tells me, 'Eat just a little bit. It's not going to hurt you. It's a party,' and so on. I tell her, 'Listen, this is what I do.'" Mara says she usually carries sugar-free candies with her so she can snack when others do, even if there's nothing suitable on the table. She tells of a friend who has had heart surgery as a result of complications of diabetes. "She doesn't care about the dieting thing. She hasn't even healed yet from her surgery, but when we were at a party she brought me a piece of cake. I told her I don't eat cake, and gave it to my husband. She said, 'I eat everything. I'm not going to diet. I just take my pills.'" Mara prefers to manage her diabetes with diet and exercise and takes no medicine for it.

Dee reports that her family is quite supportive and joins her in learning to live with diabetes. Most of her friends are supportive, too, she says, but adds, "I do have a few friends who haven't spent time learning about the disease and think that I am too restrictive." Dee doesn't argue or try to convince them; she just does what her body tells her is best.

Some people find that their diabetes management routines interfere with family routines. Grant, who depends on insulin, adjusts his insulin dose depending on what his blood glucose is at mealtime. When his family sits down to dinner, he heads for his glucose monitor, then injects his insulin. "I usually start eating my meals five minutes later than my family, after the finger stick and shot," he says. A video producer, Grant often works at home, editing tapes or doing other tasks associated with his productions; he can concentrate so deeply that he forgets to check his blood sugar and inject his insulin until after his wife announces that dinner is served. At some point he may work out a solution to this problem, such as setting an alarm to tell him it's time for his blood test and insulin, or asking his wife to warn him a few minutes before she puts dinner on the table.

Douglas, who follows a high-protein diet, finds it difficult to eat at the table with his family. "I eat differently, and as a result I often eat separately from my family, which detracts from family closeness," he says. He also believes that his dietary restrictions limit the range of social activities he can engage in with friends, and adds, "I rarely eat lunch with my colleagues anymore, which impairs my ability to strike closer relationships with them." Douglas worries that if he doesn't eat alone, he'll be tempted to eat foods that aren't good for him and feel self-conscious about eating differently from those around him. When he spoke about these problems, Douglas was only one year past his diagnosis. During that time his A1c had dropped from "the high sevens to the high fives," and he had lost forty pounds, making him a lean 203 pounds at six feet, four inches. His success at blood sugar control was sufficient motivation to keep him on the regimen he had chosen despite the way it made him uncomfortable eating with others.

Norm has made a kind of peace with his wife's sweet tooth. "She likes to bake, and it tempts me," he confesses. "If there's a blueberry cobbler in the fridge, I sneak tastes." But he insists deviations from his normal diet are under his control. "I sometimes cheat, and consciously so. On occasion I'll have a piece of cake or pie or a big bowl of pasta knowing it's going to raise my blood sugar level. When I do, I plan to be extra careful the next day, and usually am. I think it's important for my morale to cheat every so often. And though it hurts physically in that moment, a good mental attitude helps in the long term. If I was a fanatic about diet and never indulged, I'd likely give up the diet altogether and really would become frustrated about having diabetes."

Sometimes family members respond by trying to save their diabetic loved ones from themselves. Out of fear that she will develop the same complications as her diabetic relatives, Marissa's husband tries to help her control her eating. "We've had several arguments in the grocery store and in restaurants," she says. "It's an area of great difficulty and stress for me. I'm trying to be more under control myself so that he will get off my back. I just want peace, not nagging and stress." Marissa is on the right track, working to develop more self-control so her husband won't feel the need to oversee her diet. Nagging can be counterproductive. Increasing a diabetic's stress is never a good idea. Also, some people rebel at being told what to do, and fight back by eating more of what they know they shouldn't eat, just to retain a feeling of autonomy. Fortunately, while she strives to improve her diabetes management skills, Marissa has a good role model in her sister, "who is doing many things well to avoid these problems for herself. She is exercising, losing weight, and being much more responsible," Marissa says.

With refreshing honesty, Mark confesses: "My

early problems were mostly caused by the near-religious fervor of the newly diagnosed. I was very outspoken to people who invited us out that I could not be exposed to sugar in any form. I would tend to block grocery aisles while reading the ingredients label on types of food I didn't even like before I found out I was diabetic. I was pretty much not a fun guy to be around." As time went by his fanaticism disappeared. Robert, however, still struggles with this issue. He admits, "I can become kind of a bore pushing the low-carb diet if the subject of diabetes comes up."

In his talks to diabetes support groups, Gary doesn't mince words about personal responsibility. "If you're diabetic, it's great if you and your spouse can work your meals out together. But don't lay it on the one making the meals and say, 'You shouldn't have served me that. Now I feel lousy.' Well, guess what? You're the one that put it down your throat. And you've got to take responsibility for it."

DIABETES AT WORK

As many have discovered, integrating diabetes management with life outside your home can be quite a challenge. At work, schedules, workloads, and your company's culture and traditions are all factors that can become obstacles in your path toward regular, reliable blood sugar stability.

In some cases, you may be able to rely on your employer's goodwill to obtain the adjustments and accommodations you need. In the United States, unfortunately, it is no longer likely that you can invoke provisions of the Americans with Disabilities Act (ADA) to help you. A January 2002 decision by the Supreme Court now restricts ADA protection to those whose disabilities prevent them from performing one or more normal activities of daily living—cooking, bathing, feeding oneself, and so forth. It's going to be increasingly difficult to persuade an unsympathetic employer to implement the changes that can help make it easier for you to manage your diabetes. Creative thinking and good-humored assertiveness may have to substitute.

Self-employed Grant admits to some anxiety when he goes on a video shoot. "I don't have much faith in my endurance, so I filter the kinds of jobs I accept," he says. Because he's very much bothered by heat, he turns down demanding assignments in the summer. "I approach film shoots with a trepidation that I didn't feel before my diagnosis: Will I be able to move fast enough, long enough? Will we run past the six-hour limit before I need to eat a meal? If the call begins at a time that will prevent me from eating at my usual mealtime, how will I deal with it? I don't feel that I have time to test my glucose level while working, so I don't bother."

Douglas says he still struggles to eliminate periodic episodes of fatigue at work. "Currently, I experience fatigue and sleepiness every few days, for several hours during the business day. This seriously impairs my ability to work," he says. He's trying to figure out a way to have greater control over his work schedule so that he can exercise on a moment's notice to counteract changes in his blood sugar.

Alana, who works in a hospital emergency room, ran into trouble when her back was injured, making it impossible for her to move patients and stretchers. She had to switch to an assignment as an emergency room secretary, which meant working nights instead of days. "It's really had me in an uproar," she reports. "I went from working from 7 A.M. to 7 P.M. to working from 4 P.M. to 4 A.M. My whole world went upside down. It really threw me off in my eating and testing. It's one of those life decisions that I should have been more prepared for, but I didn't think of the consequences." Alana sees the irony in her situation: "I work with this every day. I tell people about stress and say that when you know high-stress things are coming up, you need to prepare yourself, you need to be ready. I guess I'm harder on myself because I feel that I should know better."

Barbara, a mental health aide, says she is very active in patient care, which makes it difficult for her to control the timing of her snacks and blood sugar testing.

Ross believes that his weight is a serious impediment at work. "Just carrying around this excess weight makes me feel uncomfortable. I'm an executive, but I don't have executive presence. I don't look slim and trim in the executive style. And if I go to a business meeting, 90 percent of the people there are not overweight, and I don't fit the norm. It sets me aside, and I feel uncomfortable." He doesn't want his coworkers to know about his condition. "Some people look at diabetes as though you're going to pass out on them, or you're going to go off the wall and have health problems. They don't recognize it as a controllable illness. They still have ancient ideas of what the disease is rather than modern knowledge of it," he explains. "And more people, including a lot of young people, are going to develop it because of their lifestyle," he adds.

Sometimes Vernon feels frustrated and ignored when his management puts out high-carbohydrate snacks that he can't eat. But, he says, "since I've stopped eating the addictive high-carb foods, I seldom get cravings. And I have my own snacks I can have when I need something—pork rinds, sunflowers seeds, and peanuts." Thad, the insurance adjuster, has a similar problem: "At work some days management orders pizza for the staff at lunchtime. I am only one out of twenty-two employees and don't want them to make everyone suffer for my sake, so I don't ask for a change in the menu or for something I can eat," he says. "If I objected to pizza, the managers might decide to stop bringing in food for the staff."

Rose, who is currently at home raising her children, wonders whether her diabetes will keep her from returning to nursing when her children are grown. She foresees three obstacles to resuming her career: "the need to be able to eat when I need to instead of when it works out for the rest of the staff, the stress of working in a hospital, and all the physical activity, which will make regulation difficult." But she remains optimistic about the future. "There are other ways of using my education," she says.

TESTING IN PUBLIC

Rose has learned to monitor her blood sugar whenever she needs to, regardless of where she is, in ways that protect her privacy and don't attract attention. For example, in a restaurant the first rule, she says, is not to put your equipment on the table, because "you don't want to upset anyone." She suggests using a napkin or tissue in your lap and doing the test there. In a movie theater it's easy to hide what you're doing because it's dark. But sometimes, Rose notes, it's just not possible to hide. "I have sat on a bench in the park and at Disney World and just tested," she says.

Using a new monitor that lets her draw blood for her test from her forearm or thigh, where the nerve endings are fewer and the pain is less, Rose has developed additional techniques to allow her to test in public without drawing attention to herself. The monitor makes a vacuum sound and then a loud click. If Rose is testing in public, she tries to do it when there is background noise. In a movie theater, for example, she will wait until the music on the sound track is loud.

"I have never gone to the bathroom to test," Rose says. "I was going to once, and my husband said he was not ashamed of what I was doing and I shouldn't be, either. I think the key to the public side of diabetes is to not get embarrassed. It is part of my life."

* * *

To be sure, learning to manage diabetes can be extremely frustrating. You have to be vigilant in starting and staying with an exercise program, changing the way you eat, and monitoring and controlling blood sugar levels on a long-term basis to avoid complications. There is no easy answer to figuring this all out. The only mistake you can make is to stop trying. If what you are doing isn't working, try something different but keep at it.

5

COMPULSIVE OVEREATING

Most of us are familiar with the phenomenon of feeling blue or anxious and finding a "comfort food" to make us feel better. If we don't experience it ourselves, we've certainly heard people we know talk about it. Entire television sitcom episodes are built around this theme. It's a human response to seek food when we're distressed. It starts at birth. The crying baby who is soothed with a breast or a bottle is learning that food is soothing. There's no way to avoid this lesson; indeed, it shouldn't be avoided, for to let a baby cry without any effort to calm him or her would be unkind, at best.

Unfortunately, the adult wish to soothe a child can lead to providing food as a response to every unpleasant situation. As we grow up, we carry our early conditioning into adulthood, and it takes a monumental effort to get beyond it. But even if we succeed, there is still the biochemical effect of too much insulin with which we must deal. We've seen that an excessive carbohydrate intake stimulates the release of too much insulin. But it is also true that too much insulin in the blood stimulates the craving for carbohydrates. And there is more to it than that. When we are under stress, we use up large amounts of the brain chemical serotonin, which is associated with mood, sleep, and appetite. When our serotonin is low, we tend to be depressed, have difficulty sleeping, and to crave food—particularly carbohydrates, which provide us with much of our serotonin. This is why people who are feeling low tend to feel better, briefly, if they feed themselves a high-carbohydrate snack. People who emphasize proteins in their diet reeducate their systems to use the amino acids in protein foods to supply them with serotonin. It may take a while (days or weeks, not months) for this learning to take effect, however. Meanwhile, they may experience depression, insomnia, and a resulting decrease in energy.

If you only occasionally eat carbohydrates for pleasure and comfort, there's no problem. But if that's your normal way of coping with psychological discomfort, the likely result is compulsive overeating. Low serotonin levels trigger hunger, and high insulin levels turn off the switch that tells you to stop eating. You may not be aware that you are eating to soothe psychological distress, but if you are pained by your relationship with food, you are probably a compulsive overeater, even if you are not overweight.

About half the people interviewed for this book identified themselves as compulsive overeaters. It's hard to say where the compulsive overeating cycle begins—with insulin resistance, which can cause temporarily low blood sugar following a high-carbohydrate meal, and lead to carbohydrate cravings; or with psychological factors—and it probably doesn't matter. No one can say for sure which influence is stronger, the chemical or psychological component. Most likely, the answer varies from person to person.

Compulsive overeating is characterized by the feeling that eating is out of control. People who eat compulsively are typically plagued by feelings of shame, disgust, and guilt. They eat whether they are hungry or not, often to the point of uncomfortable fullness. Unfortunately, people in Western society tend to see compulsive overeating as a character flaw or lifestyle choice. It isn't. It's a disease, a psychological/biochemical disturbance that should inspire compassion, not condemnation.

Many people compare compulsive overeating to binge drinking and think that both compulsive overeaters and alcoholics have some kind of deficiency in their moral fiber, that if they just got a grip on themselves, they would be cured. It's unfair to judge anyone in this way. It's especially unfair to say that the fact that some alcoholics can stop drinking is proof that a compulsive overeater can stop overeating. With sufficient determination, education, and support, an alcoholic may be able to avoid alcohol and the situations in which it is available. A compulsive eater simply cannot avoid food. Alcoholics may be able to avoid the sensory trigger that prompts them to abuse alcohol, but an overeater cannot avoid the trigger that prompts him or her to eat. Like the alcoholic, who may have cravings for life, the overeater will, too.

Compulsive overeaters aren't necessarily obsessive all the time, but when they are, they typically spend considerable mental energy thinking about food and planning what they're going to eat next. Having to deal with diabetes can wake up a sleeping compulsion because keeping blood glucose under control takes so much thought and planning. "It adds an extra problem to have to focus on food and how it's affecting your blood sugars while you're trying to break the compulsion to overeat," says Vicki. "It's tough."

It does no good to tell a binge eater to eat less. Restricting a compulsive overeater's access to food, or the choice of available foods, is apt to trigger panic—and even more compulsive overeating. To be a compulsive overeater with a diabetes diagnosis is to be vulnerable to a mixture of messages that can make you feel desperate—another trigger to compulsive overeating. Few health care practitioners can balance the conflicting requirements of the two conditions. Doctors and nutritionists are apt to emphasize blood sugar control to the exclusion of all else, overlooking the diabetic overeater's real terror of unsatisfied emotional and/or physical hunger.

CHANGING HOW YOU THINK ABOUT FOOD

Regardless of whether you take the view that the hunger is psychologically based, or that it is caused biochemically—by an imbalance of insulin and serotonin—help is available. You may want to consult a psychological counselor; you may choose to adopt the philosophy of the twelve-step group Overeaters Anonymous; you may find that the Overcoming Overeating approach appeals to you (see appendix 1 for more information); or you may choose to find your own way. Unless your life has been sufficiently threatened by diabetes to make restricting your food intake a nonissue, you're probably better off getting your eating and your blood sugar levels under control by taking an intellectually curious, investigative approach to the effect food has on your blood glucose readings.

You can reprogram your mind to conquer the negative feelings associated with compulsive overeating. When you find yourself placing values on yourself or the food you eat, tell yourself to stop thinking of yourself as "good" if you don't overeat, "bad" if you do, to stop thinking of "good" foods and "bad" ones. Stop this kind of thinking (which twelve-step groups call "stinking thinking") when you realize you're doing it. If you're in a place where no one will hear you and think you're losing it, tell yourself aloud to stop it so you not only think it but also hear yourself say it. Try this, too, when that tape starts running in your head insulting you and calling you bad names. Start thinking of eating as an activity that either accomplishes what you want to accomplish—making you feel better—or doesn't. Think about what's in your best interests—not about what makes you a "good" or "bad" person.

Compulsive overeating numbs you, but does it

really make you feel better in the long run? Do you really want to abuse yourself? Do you deserve to feel better? If you can't answer the first two questions with a heartfelt "No," and the third with an emphatic "Yes," it may be wise to talk with a mental health professional you can trust to respect your feelings about this problem. Ask the person who answers when you call to make an appointment to refer you to someone who works with people who have eating issues. Be careful not to get involved with a professional who sees obesity in moral terms. That, too, is "stinking thinking."

OVERCOMING OVEREATING WITH THE OO PROGRAM

VICKI'S STORY

Vicki is a compulsive overeater who is using the Overcoming Overeating (OO) approach to manage her diabetes. She says it helps her control the disease better than trying to follow a strict diet. Too often, dieting leads to overeating, she says. Vicki has learned to use nonjudgmental words to describe her blood sugar readings. They are *high* instead of *bad, low* instead of *good.* By testing her blood glucose after eating a variety of foods, alone and in combination, Vicki is discovering how they affect her. "I've found that many foods that most people think are totally off-limits for diabetics don't raise my blood sugars much at all, whereas foods generally considered acceptable send my sugars sky-high. I've learned it's a very individual thing," she reports.

Vicki belongs to an Internet E-mail list for compulsive overeaters. On-line, she counsels others who have been diagnosed with diabetes: "I tell them, 'Calm down. This process is going to be about reuniting with your body and your own internal signals. You'll need to do a lot of testing of your blood sugars, especially at first, so you can learn which foods affect you in what ways. Then you make adjustments without any kind of judgment or criticism.' It's very hard for somebody dealing with a compulsion to overeat to be diagnosed with diabetes. That adds an extra burden." (One technique that helps many compulsive overeaters is to find foods to binge on that don't have as drastic an effect on blood sugar levels as most starches and sugars do. For example, some people discover that eating a huge salad provides a satisfying binge.)

The story of Vicki's struggle with compulsive overeating is classic. It started when she was seven years old. Her parents put her on a weight-loss diet and soon started giving her diet pills, which are never appropriate for children and usually aren't for adults. "I wasn't even big," she recalls. "It was just what they did, so they thought I should do it, too." Thus began Vicki's twenty-five-year cycle of weight loss and compulsive overeating. After a period of dieting, she would feel so deprived that she'd lose control and eat everything in sight, beyond satiety to the point of nausea and sometimes even beyond that. "I used to sneak food through the living room while my parents were in the den watching television. I remember walking carefully because the floorboards would creak in certain places, and if I stepped on one, my dad would catch me and know I was sneaking food back to my room. I can see it was the dieting that triggered the weight problem," she says. "Every time you diet, you eventually gain more weight. It slows your metabolism and makes you want to eat more because you're sick of all the deprivation." Her perception of the disapproval of those around her probably added a psychological component to her disorder. The criticism implied by her parents' insisting that she diet to lose weight triggered—and probably still triggers—an excessive need to comfort herself.

Through her teen years, Vicki grew bigger and

bigger. She'd lose twenty-five pounds and gain thirty-five back, lose some and gain more, year after year. In her twenties she joined an Overeaters Anonymous (OA) group, a twelve-step program modeled on Alcoholics Anonymous, in which the first step was to admit she was powerless over her craving for food and then try to work herself back to "sobriety." (In the case of OA, this means reestablishing a healthy relationship with food, not, of course, abstinence from it.) By then food had become an obsession for Vicki. "I'd get up in the morning, go to a fast-food place to get breakfast, and drive to work eating in the car. When I got to work, I'd go to the cafeteria and get a small breakfast that I let everybody see me eat, so they'd think I really didn't eat much. During the day I'd get food and go into the bathroom to sneak-eat it, continuing the pattern that started when I was small."

When she was dieting, Vicki obsessed about the foods she couldn't eat: "Every waking moment, and even while sleeping, I'd think or dream about the food I wasn't letting myself have." Thinking about it now, Vicki still gets sad. She recently read diaries she wrote during her high school years. "Every single entry was about what I weighed, whether I stuck to my diet, or how I was going to do better tomorrow." When she wasn't bingeing, she was restricting her intake almost to the point of starvation. "There were days I would eat half a bowl of tomato soup and nothing more. I'd diet really hard and then binge just as hard. It was all or nothing."

Overeaters Anonymous helped, by showing her she wasn't the only person with "this horrible relationship with food," Vicki says. "It helped some with the emotional aspects, but it still triggered the rebound bingeing. I lost eighty-seven pounds in the four years I went to meetings, but the food addiction was still just as strong." OA required her to eat no more than three times a day, with no between-meal snacks. "Even if I was starving—really physically hungry—if I had eaten my three meals, I couldn't eat anything else. So there was still this external thing trying to control what I ate." That, Vicki explains, is the difference between Overeaters Anonymous and Overcoming Overeating. "OO tells me I can eat whenever I get hungry."

Vicki discovered OO by watching a television talk show on which a woman who was using that approach said she could eat two french fries and not want more because she knew she could have them whenever she wanted. "That sounded so different from my way of thinking about food that I thought, 'I've tried everything else, why not try this?'" She ordered the book that gives the program its name and forms its foundation. "When I started reading it, I was just amazed. I saw myself on every page, and it made so much sense. I could see how I got to be the size I was because of all the dieting," she says. "It took all the judgment out of it. I stopped feeling like I was some horrible monster who couldn't control herself."

Vicki's first big breakthrough came when she baked a chocolate cake. "Normally I just didn't bake because cake was something I wasn't 'supposed to have.' But I had one piece that night, and when my husband got home the next day, he was amazed that no more was gone. I had simply forgotten I had cake in the house. For me, this was a miracle."

Vicki says the only time she gains weight is when she stops the OO program and tries another approach. "I always come back to OO because it's the only thing that works for me," she says.

Overcoming Overeating teaches that there are no forbidden foods, a radical idea for someone accustomed to alternating between severe dietary restriction and rebound bingeing. For example, Vicki says, "once you realize you can have chocolate whenever you want, the urgent need to eat it right now goes away. I didn't know chocolate could go stale, but it does. Legalizing all foods and making them neutral in terms of the value we place on them is the first step—for example, chocolate is equal to lettuce, not nutritionally, but in your mind. And once that happens, after even a few weeks, you start eating from the inside instead of from external control, eating according to what your own body is wanting at the moment. And that can be salad as easily as it can be cake."

It took a while before the freedom to choose without restricting what she would eat stopped being scary, Vicki says. "Everybody thinks if you remove all restrictions, you are going to just eat and eat and never stop. Everybody thinks that until they try it. But what it does is reunite you with the inborn mechanism of feeling hungry or full that you get disconnected from when you start dieting." Still, many people do go overboard at first with this newfound freedom from restriction. OO teaches you to stock up on your favorite comfort foods so that you don't panic because they're not available when you need them. It's not surprising that compulsive overeaters will test this new availability for a while; but, according to the OO philosophy, once you get your fill, you lose interest in foods that you used to deny yourself. And when you do, Vicki says, you never regain it to the same level as before, which is why two french fries can then satisfy your desire.

Two years after she'd begun her OO journey, right after she felt she'd finally made peace with food and stopped overeating compulsively, Vicki was diagnosed with diabetes. Her first reaction was panic. "I hadn't binged in two years, and that was a miracle in itself. I thought now I'd have to change everything, go back to restricting what I could eat, and once again start fighting compulsions and cravings. I was terrified," she says. That's when Dana Armstrong, a certified diabetes educator and OO exponent, came into the picture. Jane Hirschman, one of the authors of *Overcoming Overeating,* introduced them. "Dana's the one who taught me how to implement the OO approach into diabetes," says Vicki. "It's very radical, and most doctors will look at you like you're nuts, but when my doctor saw my blood work and I was doing fine, said, 'I don't know what you're doing, but just keep doing it.'" Although her weight is still high, she reports, she's as pleased with her progress as her doctor is.

ALICE'S STORY

Alice is another binge eater who is succeeding with the OO approach. "First I tried to be the perfect patient and do everything I was supposed to do, but I couldn't sustain the dietary restrictions and ended up gaining even more weight," she says. By the time she discovered OO, she had gained a considerable amount of weight, and, she recalls, "I hated myself for not being able to control my food, even though I was trying so hard." She is now losing weight, and her blood glucose readings have gone from 315 at the time of her diagnosis to between 110 and 160, depending on where she is in relation to her last meal, the state of her stress level, and her general health. She accomplished this, Alice says, "not by dieting but by gently reminding myself that I would like to eat more healthfully." (Some people find it works best to take AA's "one day at a time" approach, but to apply it to one session of eating at a time. You might tell yourself, for example, "I choose not to abuse myself right now, but I have the option to choose to abuse myself later.") Says Alice, "I've found that when the need to take care of myself comes from an internal source, I do better than when it came from the doctor."

For Alice, fear of being scolded by her doctor about weight and eating created more stress and depression. "Stress increased my blood glucose, and depression caused me not to care about taking care of myself," she says. She found a doctor with whom she could be more comfortable. "He gives me more latitude in self-care. He doesn't yell but gently supports me, so I don't put off going in for checkups. He doesn't weigh me, which is a big relief and one of the reasons I used to put off appointments. He just asked me my weight at my first visit and now asks if there's been any significant change."

Alice still works to control the compulsion to overeat, but it doesn't come with the same irresistible force it used to do. "I used to crave sweets a lot, depending on my mood—comfort foods that are creamy and sweet, such as puddings and chocolate milk, when things were going wrong. After a big meal I would want something sweet. I used to be very fond of chocolate. Since I started working with OO, I just don't seem to need it around anymore." Using the OO technique of stocking up, Alice used to keep a big cannister filled with chocolates. After a while, she says, she just didn't care about chocolate. "My husband complained once because I wasn't keeping it filled anymore, and he liked having a little something sweet now and then, but I didn't need it. I still revert every now and then, but not very often. I just don't need it in the house, and that's been a big change. I no longer have the need to eat past full."

The OO approach, Alice says, has taught her

to tune in to what her body really wants, distinguishing between emotional eating and physiological hunger. "It's still a problem for me. When I'm tired or things are going wrong, food is my drug of choice, my way of comforting myself, but more and more I'm able to stop and ask myself if I'm really hungry or do I just need a nap. If I'm upset about something, I try just to sit with that feeling. Sometimes, because I'm in very intense psychotherapy, it's too much to sit with, and I just can't deal with the feelings. But I can tell myself it's just temporary, and until I can get through that part of therapy, there will be times when I have to eat to comfort myself. Overall I certainly eat a lot less and a lot better. I may go through an intense emotional time and eat chocolate and desserts and junk food, but pretty soon I just want vegetables and fruits and lean meats. It just happens naturally."

MAKING PEACE WITH FOOD

Most compulsive overeaters are compulsive in other ways as well. For Vicki, in the early days of having diabetes, monitoring her food intake and blood sugar became another form of compulsive activity. "At first," she says, "I became very obsessive about writing down everything I ate and testing my sugars every time I put anything into my mouth. I had to take control. I had to find out what foods helped and didn't help my blood sugars. And the only way to do it at first was to keep records. But eventually you do learn, and then you don't have to be so compulsive anymore." Vicki now has a meter that stores 250 blood glucose readings, with a link to upload the information into her computer. "I let it keep the records for me, print it out, and take it to my doctor."

Sometimes she'll look at her log between visits, but she tries not to place any judgment on how she's doing. "That's where the problems come in for me, if I start judging myself based on what the log tells me," she says. "There's no good or bad in it, only sugars that are a little high or a little low, so maybe next time I'll change the combinations of foods I eat. I keep a very neutral attitude toward it." You can also tailor the amount of testing you do according to how likely you think it is that your blood sugar needs adjusting. But even at times when your food obsession is inactive, once-a-day morning testing should be habitual.

Following a prescribed diabetic diet is tough enough for a person who isn't plagued with food cravings, but for a compulsive overeater it is nearly, if not completely, impossible. "The minute you say, 'Don't ever eat sweets because you're a diabetic, almost every diabetic starts wanting sweets even if they didn't want them before," says Vicki. "We naturally crave what's forbidden." The approach Vicki learned—and it's one that should be considered by anyone who despairs of following the conventional diabetic eating program—is to invest the time and effort necessary to learn how various foods affect their blood sugars. As important as weight loss may be in managing diabetes, seeking to lose weight when food is an obsession is apt to be futile. Instead, advises Vicki, eat what appeals to you but test your blood sugar before and after eating it and keep track of your results, without attaching value judgments to them.

This is easy to say—and extremely hard to do. If you've just been diagnosed, you're probably at least somewhat depressed and seeking comfort. Both high blood sugar and depression can impair your ability to think rationally. It may be all you can do at first to make yourself test your blood sugar and record what you've eaten, how long ago, and what your results are. But, considering the unpleasant alternatives to getting your blood sugar under control—the pain of diabetic neuropathy, the potential damage to your vision, peripheral circulation, and kidneys—keeping track of your food intake and its effect on your blood sugar is essential. Even if your goal is to manage your blood sugar without the help of medication, consider using it while you adjust to the diagnosis and learn how foods affect you. People who aren't obsessive and compulsive about food often have a hard time making the lifestyle changes diabetes requires, so it's no surprise if compulsive overeaters do, too. You may decide it's better to take medicine and not risk your health in a relapse, and work toward the day when you no longer need it.

You should do this for yourself, because you want to, because you care about yourself, and not because somebody tells you you must do it. This is a far cry from cutting your food intake in half, as Delores's doctor told her to do, or from "watching your sugars," as Gary's doctor told him.

Rose says that one of the best things she's learned is to recognize when she has overeaten, forgive herself, and move on. She sees diabetes as "a gorilla on my back. It is always there. I wake up in the morning, open my eyes, poke my finger, and my day starts by that number. It can be a pretty demanding gorilla, but I have tamed it down to a chimp. It no longer controls me; I control it. Nothing is going to remove the chimp, but my feeling of control soothes him to sleep on my back. I can maneuver through this minefield—and it is a minefield—with safety most of the time, and on tiptoes some of the time. But I can fail like anyone else. I remember standing in the kitchen, my hands on the cookie jar, tears running down my face. I want this chimp off my back so badly sometimes I can hardly stand it, but that is not going to happen today so I am content to deal with just today."

Once you make peace with food, you'll reconnect with that inner child who knew very early in life what you needed to eat and what you didn't need. And when eating is under your control, you'll have a new self-confidence that will carry over into other aspects of your life.

6

SEXUAL DYSFUNCTION

As if it weren't enough that diabetes requires you to adjust your eating habits and, often, to make other lifestyle modifications such as keeping a regular schedule when you'd rather continue functioning as a free spirit, the disease can give rise to sexual problems in both men and women. The issue is distressing to people of either sex, but it gets more attention when it happens to men, for whom dysfunction is more obvious and, unfortunately, more often a cause for embarrassment.

Estimates suggest that about half of all men who have Type 2 diabetes and are fifty years of age or older have some degree of *erectile dysfunction*, the term that has replaced in common use the demeaning term *impotence*, which more properly means inadequacy or ineffectiveness. There are no comparable statistical estimates for women, either because women are less likely than men to mention the problem during a medical visit or because doctors consider sexual dysfunction less important in women. Regardless of your sex, if you are sexually active, you should read all of the sections in this chapter—and, perhaps, ask your partner to read them as well.

NOT FOR MEN ONLY

To understand how diabetes can diminish a man's sexual functioning, one must first understand the mechanism of penile erection. When a man is stimulated sexually, blood pools in the arteries of the penis, causing it to become engorged. This increased presence of blood presses on and closes the veins that carry blood away from the penis. The process requires actions by nerves and blood vessels, both of which can be impeded by high blood sugar.

One key to penile erections is the activity of the vagus nerve, the largest nerve in the body. It runs from the brain all the way to the lower body and is the main nerve in the autonomic nervous system—the part of the nervous system that takes care of involuntary actions such as heartbeat and digestion, actions that take place without your active participation or control. Like any nerve, the vagus is subject to injury from long-term exposure to high levels of sugar in the blood. When it is damaged, it can cause more complications than any other nerve. The same vagus nerve neuropathy that causes delayed stomach emptying can also cause erectile dysfunction.

Another possible cause of erectile dysfunction is fatty deposits in the arteries that provide for penile engorgement. Insulin resistance, the underlying cause of most cases of Type 2 diabetes, often causes high levels of blood fats as well. The buildup of cholesterol in the blood vessels, known as peripheral vascular disease, can cause not only heart attacks and strokes but also constriction of the arteries that bring blood to the penis. People who have diminished circulation in their legs are most apt to have this problem as well.

Insulin resistance by itself can cause erectile dysfunction. The inner surface of the heart and blood vessels is lined with a silky coating of cells called the endothelium. One important function of the endothelium is production of nitric oxide (not to be confused with nitrous oxide, which is laughing gas). Nitric oxide helps determine whether blood vessels will relax or tighten.

Arteries become constricted in the absence of nitric oxide, restricting the flow of blood. This is a cause of high blood pressure. When the endothelium of the blood vessels in the penis doesn't make enough nitric oxide, erectile dysfunction can result. Insulin is essential to the production of nitric oxide. In Type 2 diabetes, the endothelium resists insulin's message to produce normal amounts of nitric oxide, arteries impede the free flow of blood, and erection is compromised.

High blood sugar alone can cause erectile dysfunction by depriving the diabetic man of libido, or sexual desire. Testosterone, a male hormone (also present in females, but in lower concentrations), is the chemical messenger of sexual desire. High blood sugar drives down testosterone levels, decreasing libido and resulting in at least temporary erectile dysfunction.

Sexual stimulation is more than a mechanical function; the mind and emotions are also involved. The fear and uncertainty that often accompany the diagnosis of diabetes can deal a crushing blow to a man's ego, making him feel vulnerable at first and robbing him of self-confidence. Sometimes all it takes for erectile dysfunction to develop, particularly in a man whose self-confidence is weakened, is one episode in which he fails to achieve an erection—a common enough occurrence even among men who don't have diabetes—and this failure is apt to trigger anxiety the next time the opportunity presents itself. Sufficient anxiety stimulates the production of adrenal stress hormones, which interfere with erection, and a vicious cycle begins: An erection failure leads to fear of a recurrence, which leads to another erection failure, and so on. This can happen to any man; what makes it worse in a man with diabetes is the added fear that it is a sign that the diabetes is out of control. "You have to realize that when you're first getting into diabetes, you're afraid of everything. There's a definite fear factor," says Gary.

There are ways to avoid the onset of erectile dysfunction and to relieve it if it has already occurred. First, it's important to understand that the problem is related to how high blood sugar levels have been and for how long. There's no absolute rule on how high an individual's blood sugar levels would have to be or for how long to cause the dysfunction. What is known, however, is that getting your blood sugar to a level that you and your doctor agree is good for you—and keeping it there—will improve your ability to achieve and maintain an erection. It may take weeks, it may take a year or more, but there is no reason to give up just because your sugar levels are high now and you are experiencing erectile dysfunction. Perhaps understanding the relationship between high blood sugar and erectile dysfunction is what you need to motivate yourself to take control over your diabetes.

Smoking or using smokeless tobacco products can compound a diabetic's problems achieving an erection. In the short term, tobacco constricts blood vessels, including those that bring blood to the penis. In the long term, it damages blood vessels, causing problems that are hard to reverse. But reverse them you can, if you stop using tobacco. Give your body a chance, and its natural healing processes will work in your favor.

Some prescription medications, especially some mood-altering drugs and blood pressure pills, can interfere with the ability to have an erection. If you suspect that a drug you are taking is involved in this problem, discuss alternative medications with your doctor. Usually you can find a substitute that won't have this effect. If you have high blood pressure, you may be able to work toward bringing it down to the point where you no longer need any drug to control it. In Rand's case, he did have an erection, but it was painful. It turned out that the type of diabetes drug he was taking can sometimes cause this problem.

If you can handle alcohol, a small amount—a glass of red wine, consumed in a leisurely manner, for example—may help you and your blood vessels to relax. People who depend on insulin should not consume alcohol, because it can either increase or decrease the insulin's effect. Large quantities of alcohol will interfere with some diabetes medications, but your doctor will probably say a single drink is acceptable. Of course, if you cannot stop after one drink, this is not a good idea for you. Usually, a small amount of alcohol will have little or no effect on your blood sugar, but you should test yourself once or twice a half hour to an hour after taking a drink to be sure this is true for you. And keep in mind that large amounts of alcohol can kill all chances for an erection even in men who don't have any health problems.

One of the benefits of regular exercise, beyond its ability to make cells more sensitive to the insulin your pancreas produces, is that it stimulates the development of capillaries, the tiny vessels that supply your tissues with blood. The more carrying capacity you have for your blood, the more likely you will be to achieve an erection.

There are also mechanical and chemical ways that can help overcome erectile dysfunction. The drug sildenafil (Viagra) is the best-known, but not the only, option. Taken about an hour before intercourse is to occur, Viagra helps more than half the men who try it, so it's worth discussing with your doctor. It works by enhancing the effects of nitric oxide in relaxing the blood vessels of the penis. Since nitric oxide is released in response to sexual stimulation, manual foreplay becomes more important than it normally is for most men. Norm is one Viagra success story. He says, "I'm grateful for Viagra as well as to [former U.S. senator] Bob Dole for being open about it." However, if you have a heart condition and are using nitroglycerine, Viagra is not for you. The combination of sildenafil and nitrates can cause a drop in blood pressure that can be fatal.

If Viagra fails, there are other options. One of the most popular is a vacuum erection device—an "Erector set," as some men call it. This device has three components: a plastic tube, a pump, and a rubber ring. You operate it by first placing the tube over your penis; then you use the attached pump—hand- or battery-operated—to pull blood into your penis, which results in erection; finally, you slide the ring over the tube and onto the base of your penis, then remove the tube. Most makers of such devices warn that the ring, which prevents blood from flowing out of the penis, will make the penis cold to the touch and must not be left in place for more than an hour. It takes a bit of practice to become skilled at using this device, but its success doesn't depend on emotional factors and isn't hampered by vagal neuropathy, so it's worth considering.

Men who can achieve an erection but have difficulty maintaining it may find useful a penile constriction ring, similar to those used with the vacuum device but available separately. When you get an erection, you put the ring at the base of your penis (it stretches to allow you to put it into place) and remove it immediately after intercourse. With the vacuum erection device and the constriction ring, it is sometimes advisable to cut or shave the pubic hair for a quarter inch or so around the base of the penis.

Other mechanical devices, known as penile prostheses, exist. One is a bendable, semirigid rod that is surgically implanted into the penis. The other is a system of inflatable cylinders, activated by a pump surgically placed within the scrotum. The pump is activated by compressing a bulb in the scrotum when an erection is wanted. Both devices, because they require surgery, carry with them the risk of infection and mechanical malfunction. Fixing the malfunction usually means another surgical procedure, so these options are less popular than the noninvasive pump system.

There are two more chemical alternatives. One is injection of a drug such as phentolamine or papaverine into the penis. This causes blood to be drawn into the penis, causing an erection. The needle used for these injections is so fine that most men find it only minimally unpleasant. Usually, this method is prescribed by a urologist, who will teach you how to administer the injection and monitor your success in one or more office visits. You'll need instruction, too, to learn to use the last option currently available. Called the MUSE system, it consists of a device containing a small plunger with which you insert a tiny pellet of medication, prostaglandin, into the penis. This causes the arteries of the penis to relax so that more blood can flow in and an erection can result. As with Viagra, the stimulation of foreplay is useful to enhance this effect.

Another common problem among men with diabetes is retrograde ejaculation, in which seminal fluid moves in the wrong direction. Instead of coming out of the penis at the time of orgasm, semen is propelled backward and absorbed by the body. While the result can be both surprising and alarming, it presents a problem only for a man who is trying to father a child. Medically, it seems to present no danger of long-term complications. If fertility is not an issue, the best thing to do is ignore it. If you're trying to have a child, it's a matter for discussion with a urologist. In most cases, it can be successfully treated.

NOT FOR WOMEN ONLY

Sexual response in both men and women depends on genital engorgement. So the health of nerve fibers and blood vessels in the genitals is just as important to a woman's sexual functioning as it is to a man's. Nevertheless, malfunction of the female genitals—the clitoris, vulva, and vaginal wall—may be less obvious to a woman's partner than erectile dysfunction is to a man's. As this is being written, studies are under way to find out whether Viagra can be helpful to women, since nitric oxide plays the same role in genital engorgement in women as it does in men. Early results are promising.

Neuropathy can cause loss of sensation in the genital area, reducing sexual arousal and pleasure. Loss of arousal means decreased blood flow into the area. It also means decreased lubrication of the vaginal wall, which can lead to pain and irritation. Says Grace, who is forty-nine years old, "Having relations can be hard. You have vaginal dryness, and you just don't get in the mood most of the time. It's really annoying." Grace talked with her doctor about this problem. "He's given me creams and different stuff to use. I know it's from the diabetes, because before that, I was fine."

If dryness is a problem, you can find a variety of vaginal lubricants at any good drugstore. Most lubricants are odorless and tasteless so as not to get in the way of free sexual expression. Like the devices that aid men with erection problems, these products do detract a bit from the spontaneity of sexual activity, but usually they're not so intrusive as to ruin the experience.

Loss of libido plays as important a role in women's sexuality as it does in men's. Libido gets you in the mood to be aroused. Arousal causes the vaginal sphincter—the ringlike muscle at the opening to the vagina—to relax so that penile penetration is not uncomfortable. If the sphincter doesn't relax, intercourse is likely to be painful. Many women find they can learn to make the sphincter loosen by concentrating on it and squeezing the muscle as though trying to resist urinating. Lie on your back, squeeze, and let loose a few times. It takes practice, but you can do it.

In general, women are even more sensitive than men to feelings of being unattractive and undesirable. Having diabetes, as well as being overweight, can exacerbate those feelings. Western society's ideal for feminine beauty is impossible—and, in many cases, unhealthy—for most women to achieve. If, in addition, your body image has depended on considering yourself physically fit, it takes some time and self-talk—perhaps with the help of a psychological counselor—to adapt to the fact that you're not a perfect physical specimen. Says Roberta, "Somewhere deep inside, now that I have this disease, I don't feel very desirable to my husband." She knows this isn't related to her husband's attitude. "It's all in my head; he is very helpful and supportive. But sometimes your own thoughts get in the way, and at times you no longer feel good enough."

Depression is a powerful deterrent to sexuality. It's all wrapped up with feelings of loss, inadequacy, unattractiveness, and, perhaps, insecurity. In a long-standing relationship in which the woman's illness shifts the focus from her husband's needs to her own, there may be anxiety that he won't accept the change. Women often get less support from their doctors for sexual dysfunction than do men. In one small survey published in a diabetes journal, it was reported that 85 percent of physicians said they routinely asked diabetic men about sexual difficulties, but only 33 percent routinely asked women. Of course, you don't have to wait to be asked. You may have been raised to be modest, and you may find it particularly difficult to discuss sex if your doctor is a man, but if sex has been an important part of your committed relationship, it's worth the effort to work up your courage and bring up the subject yourself. One way to do this is to try role-playing first with a close female friend. Ask her to play the doctor's part, and you take the role of the patient. Or, if that's too hard the first time, pretend you are the doctor and she is the patient. You don't have to use real details when you start this role-playing exercise; you only have to bring up the subject and practice talking about it, using the accepted medical terms for your genitals and your partner's until you can say them without embarrassment. The process is called *desensitization*, and it almost always works.

For women as well as men, the best way to overcome sexual dysfunction is to get blood sugar levels under control. High blood sugar reduces energy and vitality, making you less receptive to sex. Nerve damage and poor circulation can be reversed to a considerable extent—how much depends on how high your blood glucose has been and for how long. High blood sugar also increases the occurrence of vaginitis, yeast infections, and urinary tract infections, all of which can cause sexual dysfunction even if their symptoms are mild.

Tobacco and alcohol also can interfere with sexual responsiveness. Drugs, especially some blood pressure medications and antidepressants, can cause problems. Antianxiety and antidepression drugs can increase vaginal dryness or blunt your ability to respond to any emotional stimulus, including sexual arousal. If you suspect your medications are interfering with your sexual pleasure, mention this to your doctor. There are almost always alternatives. If you don't ask your doctor, chances are your doctor won't ask you.

THE IMPORTANCE OF SEX

If diabetes has impeded your sex life, consult your health professional and communicate openly with your partner. Getting your blood sugar under control is the primary prerequisite to restoring sexual vitality.

Sexuality is an important part of life, regardless of your age, but there are many ways to express it. If diabetes or any other condition makes having intercourse or achieving orgasm a problem, don't forget that hugging, kissing, snuggling, even affectionate remarks are all aspects of sexual expression. What matters is that you love and feel loved by your partner.

If one partner has become sexually dysfunctional because of diabetes, that's the time that the other person's loving reassurance becomes crucial, both to the health of your relationship and to the ultimate success of the partner with the sexual problem in coming back to full functioning. A failure of sexual performance is much like falling off a horse. The only way to overcome your fear is to get back on the horse, to try again as soon as possible. But trying takes courage and encouragement. Sex therapists suggest that one way to get around the performance anxiety that often follows an encounter that didn't work out the way you hoped it would is to agree that the next lovemaking session will not include intercourse, but only whatever form of stroking and stimulation appeals to both of you. Remove orgasm as the goal, and focus on giving each other comfort and pleasure. You may be pleasantly surprised at how the experience turns out.

And while you're enjoying each other without requiring any specific outcome, spend some of your out-of-bed time thinking and talking about how the diabetic partner can further the goal of normalizing blood sugar, which may solve the problem that interferes with full sexual performance—and what the nondiabetic partner can do to help. Sex is a team activity; managing diabetes can be, too.

7

FROM STRUGGLE TO SUCCESS

Type 2 diabetes is a single disease that expresses itself in each individual in a slightly different way. Heredity is probably the major factor in determining which foods cause blood sugar spikes and which do not. Joseph, who lives in British Columbia, is half Native American and half Scots-Irish; he says he apparently inherited his metabolism from the native side of the family, because he doesn't get blood sugar spikes from corn, but he does from wheat. He attributes this to the fact that for his native ancestors corn was a major component of their diet, but wheat was not.

When people at support groups get around to talking about how different foods affect them, one person will say, "I can eat rice, but I can't eat potatoes, because rice leaves me nice and level, but potatoes make me spike." And then the next person will say exactly the opposite.

Then there's the fact that what is low blood glucose for one person is a triumph in control for another. Sylvia's blood sugar levels have been so high for so long that, she says, a blood glucose of 120 would make her faint from hypoglycemia, so she carries glycogen with her to counteract her insulin when her blood sugar starts to go too low. Debra's evening blood glucose depends as much on when she ate her dinner as on what she ate. By contrast, for some people who, like Debra, do not depend on insulin, an hour's delay in a meal is either not important or would cause low, not high, blood sugar.

Some people find it easier to control their blood sugar on a low-carbohydrate diet. But even though Raymond was raised on such a diet, he became diabetic anyway. Paul sums it up using a common Internet expression. "Always remember YMMV [Your Mileage May Vary]," he says. "In diabetic terms, that means that Dick may get away with eating a cup of rice, while Jane will see her blood glucose go up by 300 points from that same serving."

Some diabetics view oral medications as a way to eat more of their favorite foods without paying a blood-glucose penalty. On the other hand, people like Mara want to avoid medicines as long as they can. "I know there are diabetics who take medicines three times a day so they can have their little plates full. I like it better the other way, where I control my diabetes by what I eat and don't eat," she says. Such decisions are entirely up to you. Your family and friends have the right to encourage you to take good care of yourself, but nobody has the right to tell you what to do.

While much is known about Type 2 diabetes in general, when it comes to the unique individual that is you, there is a great deal to learn, and you're the one who has to learn it. You can choose to see having diabetes as an adventure in which you have the opportunity to enhance your prospects for a long and rich life. If you approach mealtimes and blood glucose tests with curiosity and a desire to learn, you stand a good chance of being a diabetes success story.

Not one of the people who was interviewed for this book claims to have all the answers, but all have made peace with their situation and are committed to continuing to learn and manage their disease in a way that will let them live as full and healthy a life as possible. In this chapter, a number of them respond to the question "What advice would you give to someone around your age [i.e., a Baby Boomer] who has just been diagnosed?" As you will see, some advice contradicts other advice—particularly when it comes to what to eat and what to avoid—but there is a common thread running through it all: Stay calm, learn as much as you can, and make a firm commitment to take good care of yourself.

ATTITUDE IS EVERYTHING

Your attitude toward the situation in which you find yourself will be a major factor, perhaps the most important one, in determining how successful you are in handling it. Grant says it's important at the outset to let yourself experience the natural feelings that come with bad news. "Let the fact of your diagnosis sink in," he says. "Let your feelings about it come—anger, grief, dread, fear—whatever they may be." They're all valid feelings, and if you push them away too quickly, they'll lurk in the shadows to haunt you and obstruct your path to success. And, says Carl, "if you're going to go through denial, do it quickly and then get help. Do whatever it takes to be as well as you can be. You owe it to yourself not to spend your later days regretting the medical complications that might not have been if you'd gotten a handle on it early in the game." Vicki offers words of caution—and comfort: "Take [diabetes] seriously; don't mess around with it. But at the same time, don't fret and worry about it. That will only make things worse. Don't let fear take over. You can control it, and you can live a normal life." Margaret agrees: "Don't be afraid. Fear is the worst possible feeling you can have when you're first diagnosed." She adds, "Most of all, keep a positive attitude. It's difficult, but in the long run it pays to look at your life in a positive way."

"Don't panic or despair," says Delores. "It's not that big a thing, really. You just have to remember that you are the person in charge of your health; it's in your hands to control the diabetes, not your doctor's. The better you get at controlling those after-meal blood glucose spikes, the less you have to worry about the awful complications of diabetes."

Adjusting to the fact that you have diabetes will be easier if you don't fight against it, advises Elaine. "Your life will change, in some cases more than in others, but you can learn to handle it. Try not to think of the change as having to suffer; that will only make you miserable and make it harder for you to adjust." She adds, "Remember that diabetes is not your fault. You may have done—or not done—things that made it more likely to happen, but don't forget that others have behaved the same way and don't have diabetes. There's much more to it than just your lifestyle in the past."

"This is a new beginning," says Rose. "Now you know why you have been feeling so crummy. Now you can find out what to do about it." Rose also counsels calm: "Take a deep breath. Life will go on. It will change, but it will go on."

Marissa offers the following advice: "Don't let yourself get overwhelmed. Don't expect too much progress too soon. Make small changes, and they'll gradually add up to a big difference. Respect your individual differences. Remember that what works for one person won't necessarily work for you."

Roberta has learned that there are some things she can't change but must simply accept. "My goal is to always be able to say 'I'm doing the best I can'—not 'I'm trying to do the best I can.' You can't 'try' with this disease. You have to 'do.'" Roberta says it's important to be patient and treat yourself as you'd treat a good friend. "This can't be corrected overnight. You really have to work at it. Be sensible, be honest with yourself, and acknowledge your feelings. Be patient with yourself, find joy in all you do, and love yourself."

Barbara adds, "Don't ever give up. There is a right way for everyone to get their diabetes under control, but if you stop searching, you'll never find your personal means to success."

KNOWLEDGE IS POWER

You don't have to be a genius to be able to learn what you need to know to manage your diabetes. You're already the world's foremost authority when it comes to your own body. Nobody knows it the way you do, from the inside out. If you're not used to paying close attention to how you react to various triggers—food and stress, for the most part—now that you know how important it is to do that, you will begin to do so, almost automatically. You'll notice how you feel in relation to what you've eaten and what's going on in your life. Then you'll begin to gain a working knowledge of your blood sugar levels—by using your glucose monitor and keeping records—and process additional information gained from the experience of others. You may want to understand the mechanics of diabetes—how food metabolism works in general and how it affects blood sugar levels in people with diabetes—or you may not want to explore this subject in depth. The choice is a matter of personal preference. But you owe it to yourself and those who care about you to use your inborn intelligence about your own body, and that's something everyone can do, regardless of education or IQ.

The knowledge you obtain from testing your blood glucose levels is invaluable. "Write everything down so you can see the patterns develop," advises Rose. "The effort you invest in yourself will pay you back handsomely." Norm has advice for people who are reluctant to test their blood sugar frequently: "Turn the monitoring into a game or a challenge—anything that appeals to you. I look at it as a sporting event. Others might make it into a game of poker. Do what works for you."

One of the benefits of regular testing is that you may be surprised at what you can eat without undesirable effects, says Vernon, who grieved at first for the high-sugar, high-starch foods he'd never be able to eat again. He soon found through testing that while some foods were inappropriate for him, he could replace them with others he likes quite well. "Check your blood sugar regularly," he says. "Don't believe it when it seems like you can't eat anything you like anymore. Do believe that there are addicts to foods that are high in starches, and you are probably one of them. The good news is that you can get out of the addictive cycle, and the cravings will stop. Plus, there are still many delicious things you can eat."

Learning about diabetes, says Mark, "is your responsibility, and in the end, it's you that sinks or swims." Others echo his call for self-reliance. "Insist on some training from a certified diabetes educator and take charge of your own diabetes," advises Vicki. "Learn all you can and don't just blindly trust your doctor. The doctor isn't the one who will have physical complications arise if your diabetes isn't controlled—you will."

Elaine emphasizes the value of learning as much as you can as a way to relieve the stress of being diagnosed with diabetes. "It will help ease your fears," she says, and recommends seeing a certified diabetes educator and a diabetic nutritionist. "They will work with you to help get you headed in the right direction."

Gary likens diabetes management to the "one day at a time" philosophy that has come into our culture through Alcoholics Anonymous. However, with diabetes, he says, "it's more like one hour at a time. What you're doing now is going to affect you two to three hours from now. That's where the fear really comes in, because unless you're really educated about it, you don't know that. So you eat something that doesn't sit right with your blood sugars, and in another couple of hours you're going to feel pretty lousy. That's the difference between going on a diet to lose weight and controlling diabetes so you feel well all the time. You learn to eat correctly to avoid those bad feelings."

Mark encourages you to "ask your doctor questions and listen to the answers. Write them down if you need to. Remember, the only stupid questions are the ones you don't ask." If you suffer from more that one ailment, he suggests that you "talk to your physician about the team approach to your diabetes. Most doctors are pleasantly surprised with patients that take an active interest in their treatment, so make your physician happy and be part of the team."

For many people with diabetes, joining a support group yields great benefits. Most hospitals sponsor diabetes support groups. Internet groups provide an alternative to face-to-face meetings. Some people are more comfortable with a higher level of anonymity, and they can contact the on-line group anytime they wish, regardless of the hour or day, without having to wait for a regularly scheduled meeting. (There is a list of on-line diabetes support groups in appendix 1.) Walter says, "Get into a support group and vent there. Other members understand what you're going through and that sometimes you need a shoulder to lean on. After I found my group, I didn't feel so alone."

Among the things you'll learn in an on-line support group, which is more independent of a hospital's treatment philosophy, is that there are many different approaches, and that no single approach works for everyone. "There is the low-carb diet versus the ADA diet; insulin versus oral medications versus doing it all with diet and exercise. Keep an open mind and try different things, until you find what works for you," says Delores.

Barbara, an enthusiastic exponent of Internet groups, notes that "there are many sites with legitimate information and support for individuals with diabetes. If you have access to the Internet, use it to your advantage." If you don't have a computer in your home, your local library can help you to get on-line, and you'll have professional guidance in how to search for what you need. Barbara continues, "There are lots of online magazines, diabetic recipes, information on home glucose testing and equipment, and so forth. The list is absolutely endless! Let me put it this way: If knowledge is power, then the Internet can make you a superhero."

WORDS OF INSPIRATION

It's normal and understandable, before you've found the keys to controlling your own unique case of diabetes, to think your life is changed forever for the worse; to mourn the loss of spontaneity; to miss the freedom you once had to eat whatever you felt like eating whenever you felt like eating; and to resent the need to discipline yourself to exercise, test your blood sugars, and keep records. Nobody who understands the changes diabetes makes in your life can look down on you if you feel like complaining. But if you take your disease seriously and determine not to let it beat you down, even if you never come to be glad you have diabetes, before long you will find the good parts of it, as the individuals quoted here have done.

For people with a chronic, incurable illness, experienced diabetics can be a quite positive group. Roberta, who admits to some continuing struggles, says nevertheless, "I'm getting the hang of this, and I will be fine. I've lost over thirty pounds that really needed to come off. I get out every day and walk, and where I walk is beautiful—birds and wildlife, ponds and fields, all the things I was missing before diabetes."

Charles points out, "If you must have diabetes, this is the best time so far. There are substitutes for almost every kind of high-sugar food. Opportunities for good health have never been greater. I'm healthier than I've felt for a long, long time." Thad agrees: "I'm probably healthier now than at any time in my life. I ran fifteen miles a couple of days ago; I couldn't have done that a few months ago. I've probably extended my life because now I eat healthier foods and have gotten my weight down to a healthy place. Diabetes can be controlled, and it can cause your life to be longer—not just seem longer—because it gets you focused on what is important for your health."

Others express satisfaction with their lives. Walter: "I have a good life. If having diabetes is the worst thing to happen to me and my family, then that's fine with me." Mark: "Diabetes is not the end of your life, unless you ignore it and let it control your life and activities." Robert: "My life is just fine as it is. I'm satisfied with what I eat, and in general, things are good." Barbara: "For the first time in years, I'm actually quite satisfied with my life."

Raymond sees his diabetes diagnosis as a blessing. "I'm taking better care of myself now than I would have if I weren't diagnosed," he says. "After forty years of smoking, I quit, not because my health was failing, but because it was still good and I decided I'd pushed my luck as far as I wanted to push it. So my attitude is that being diagnosed was not a hardship because it led me to look at my health and do everything possible to be as well as I can be." He adds, "I have a wife-to-be who's nine years younger than I am. She made me promise that I'm going to live longer than she will. And I'll keep that promise, whatever it takes."

Elaine also thinks of being diagnosed with diabetes as "probably the best thing that could have ever happened." She explains: "Being rather lacking in energy because of other [chronic] illnesses, I was very inclined to eat whatever was easiest. Often that meant making a big pot of something and eating it for several days, in whatever quantity happened to land on my plate. No vegetables for two weeks? No problem, as long as there was enough of something else to fill me up. Even now, I don't always eat balanced meals, but they are much closer to being balanced. Less fat, less salt, and controlled portions—and I'm eating lots more vegetables."

Diabetes isn't only about food, though, says Elaine. "A lot of it is the psychological aspect. Chronic illnesses take away so much, sometimes it feels like they steal my very soul, and most certainly it feels as if they strip away control of my life because I never know just how I will feel when I am trying to plan ahead. But even though diabetes is chronic, I can take pride in having learned to be in control. Some days I have less control than others and one more piece of pizza calls rather loudly, but I'm still in control, for I have made a conscious choice. I would not have wished for diabetes, but it is something I can live with."

Speaking at the support group meeting where he stepped into his old, tentlike trousers, Gary says, "Every diabetic has to make a decision. Mine was to turn a negative into a positive, and that's what I do every day even now to keep me from thinking that that doughnut looks like a good idea." He concludes, "Everybody knows what the repercussions are from diabetes. The bottom line is, you can lead a good life. It's probably the second best thing that ever happened to me. Getting married was the first. My life is really changed—for the better. You're always going to get obstacles thrown at you; diabetes is just another obstacle. But once you overcome it, you're going to feel that much better because you've got everything under control."

EPILOGUE

WHAT LIES AHEAD

The good news about the upsurge in cases of Type 2 diabetes is that the disease has caught the attention of medical researchers and technology companies eager to provide new products and services to help people control their blood sugar.

Blood sugar monitoring will become easier and the pain will be gone with the advent of a new generation of glucose meters that use interstitial fluid, found between cells in the skin, instead of blood as the testing sample. A variety of devices will reach the market between 2004 and 2006. Some will use tiny laser beams or near-infrared light rays to create pores in the skin and obtain interstitial fluid for testing; others will use a patch to attract the fluid. Several such devices are being developed and tested as this is being written. In the United States, they will need to be approved by the Food and Drug Administration, which is a lengthy and painstaking process. As is true with all new technologies, these devices will probably be quite expensive (in the hundreds of dollars) when they are first released, but prices will decrease sharply once the makers have earned back their development costs.

Coming on the market in the near future are kits for testing your HbA1c at home, instead of the doctor's office, although these kits will probably require a doctor's prescription. One kit consists of a lancet, a card on which to place the resulting blood sample, and a mailer to send the sample to a laboratory. Another uses a device much like a glucose meter that accepts a blood sample and yields a reading in eight minutes.

Also on the way are new methods for delivering insulin, which is currently available only by injection. Of the 16 million Type 2 diabetics in the United States today, about 3 or 4 million use insulin. Experts say doctors are reluctant to prescribe it for Type 2 because so many people fear needles. So far, pharmaceutical company researchers have been unable to find any way of getting insulin into the body without puncturing skin. But work is under way to develop an insulin pill that can be absorbed in the digestive system, as well as an inhalable insulin that can be absorbed in the lungs, the way asthma medication is. Even closer to release, though, is a device that sprays insulin into the mouth. This simple and compact device looks much like an asthma inhaler. It may well be on the market by the time you read this book.

Also watch for a device that can be implanted under the skin to monitor blood sugar levels automatically and deliver the right amount of insulin into the bloodstream without any action on the part of the user. It uses a kind of gel that swells when it contacts a glucose molecule. When it swells, it releases a minute amount of insulin. The device is self-regulating; insulin is released only when it is needed. You can expect to hear more about this in 2005 or 2006.

Pharmaceutical companies are developing new drugs that will work in the ways current drugs do, only better. By 2004 we should see a third generation of pills that improve the body's ability to use its own insulin, increase insulin secretion, or decrease the liver's output of glucose, sometimes in combinations of two or all three of these functions.

Experiments are under way using an intestinal hormone called glucagon-like-peptide-1 (GLP-1), which stimulates the production and secretion of insulin in the pancreas and tends to lower blood glucose. People with Type 2 diabetes are deficient in GLP-1. The GLP-1 used in the experiments is short-acting and must be injected, but researchers are trying to develop a long-acting form that can be delivered in a pill. In a small study GLP-1 was found to decrease HbA1c by 1.3 percent in six weeks. Four companies are racing to get GLP-1 on the market.

Another promising investigation revolves around ghrelin, a stomach hormone that stimulates the secretion of growth hormone and, at the same time, decreases insulin levels and increases glucose levels. Researchers are working on a medication that will inhibit the release of ghrelin, hoping to overcome its effects on insulin levels and blood sugar in Type 2 diabetics. The results of this work are probably several years off.

For people with debilitating diabetic neuropathy, an effective, noninvasive way to increase the supply of nitric oxide, hence improving circulation to nerves and blood vessels, is newly available, but little known. Called the Anodyne Therapy System (ATS), it uses near-infrared light that penetrates tissues and increases blood flow, healing skin ulcers quickly and improving nerve function.

From the insurance industry comes a program called diabetes management that holds the promise of being a win-win situation for both patients and insurers. If your health insurance plan enrolls you in diabetes management, you are assigned a nurse or diabetes educator who keeps in touch with you by phone, answering your questions and encouraging you to follow the treatment plan your doctor has recommended. Think of it as having your mother check in periodically to make sure you're taking good care of yourself. The idea of having someone remind you to eat right, exercise, take your medicine, and see the doctor for regular checkups may seem intrusive, but patients in diabetes management programs turn out to lose fewer days of work and live more active, enjoyable lives. Of course, health insurance companies pay for the service because it saves them money by reducing the number of hospital admissions and emergency room visits.

Diabetes management may soon be combined with telemedicine, providing you with a device that attaches to your telephone or computer. You place your finger in the device to have your blood glucose read from interstitial fluid and transmitted to your diabetes manager or physician.

Even with all these advances, the course of Type 2 diabetes, more than any other disease, will continue to depend on the patient. Experts say that for every percentage point you can shave off your HbA1c, you reduce the risk of damaging complications by 25 percent. One point on the HbA1c equals thirty points on your glucose meter. Diet and exercise are the keys to glucose management. What you eat and whether you exercise are up to you, not your doctor. Health care professionals are there to educate and support you, but they can't make your lifestyle choices for you. You are in charge of your condition.

GLOSSARY

A1c. See HbA1c.

Carbohydrates. Chains of sugar molecules found in breads and cereals, pasta, grains, vegetables, fruits, most dairy products, and sweets.

C-peptide. A small protein that is a by-product of insulin production. The C-peptide test measures the amount of this protein in the blood, revealing how much insulin a person's pancreas is producing. Type 1 diabetics do not have any C-peptide unless they are taking insulin. The test is also used to determine whether a person is taking sufficient insulin.

Diabetic coma. A condition associated with extremely high blood sugars (usually more than 1,000). Early symptoms are dehydration, confusion, and drowsiness. Loss of consciousness and even death may occur. Treatment involves fluid replacement and insulin injections to reduce the blood sugar level.

Diabetic ketoacidosis. See *Ketoacidosis*.

Diabetic neuropathy. See *Neuropathy*.

Erectile dysfunction. Also called impotence. The inability to achieve or sustain an erection of the penis. May be caused by neuropathy, circulatory problems, psychological problems, or a combination of these.

Food pyramid. A guide to daily food intake developed by the American Dietetic Association and promoted by the U.S. Department of Agriculture. Depicted as a pyramid with carbohydrates at its base, this guide recommends that 55 to 60 percent of calories should come from carbohydrate sources (grains, starches, and sugars), and no more than 30 percent from fats, leaving 20 to 25 percent of caloric intake to proteins.

Gastroparesis. A condition of delayed stomach emptying; one of the complications of diabetes.

Glucagon. A hormone released by the alpha cells of the pancreas in response to too little glucose in the bloodstream. Also a medication used by insulin-dependent diabetics to overcome hypoglycemia.

Glucose. A simple sugar that results from the breakdown of foods in the body; normally, the body's main source of energy.

Glucose monitor. A device for checking blood glucose (blood sugar) levels.

Glycemic index. A scale that shows how rapidly various foods release glucose into the bloodstream.

Glycogen. Glucose stored in the liver and released when blood sugar levels drop too low.

HbA1c. A blood test that gives an average blood glucose reading for the preceding two or three months.

Hormone. A chemical, released by a gland, that carries information or instructions to some part of the body.

Hyperglycemia. High blood sugar.

Hypoglycemia. Low blood sugar.

Insulin. A hormone released by the beta cells of the pancreas in response to glucose in the bloodstream. Type 1 diabetics do not produce insulin and must obtain it by injection. A small percentage of Type 2 diabetics use insulin as well, usually by choice because it allows more flexibility in dietary choices.

Insulin resistance. A condition in which the cells of the body do not accept insulin's instruction to store glucose for future use as energy; a leading cause of Type 2 diabetes.

Ketoacidosis. A dangerous complication of diabetes, caused by extremely high blood sugar brought about by a lack of insulin or severe insulin resistance. The blood becomes highly acidic, and normal metabolic processes are disturbed. Ketoacidosis is very rare in Type 2 diabetes. It is not the same as ketosis.

Ketones (also ketone bodies). A by-product of the breakdown of free fatty acids; a source of energy.

Ketosis. The condition in which ketones provide energy in preference to glucose. In nondiabetics and diet-controlled Type 2 diabetics the pancreas prevents ketosis from becoming ketoacidosis.

Libido. Sexual interest, desire.

Neuropathy. Dysfunction of a nerve; diabetic neuropathy results from nerve damage caused by high blood sugar.

Protein. Found in animal and plant foods, proteins provide energy and the amino acids necessary for tissue growth and repair.

R-to-R interval study. A medical test that records the peaks and valleys of the heartbeat; an indicator of vagus nerve function.

Serotonin. A neurotransmitter (brain chemical) associated with appetite, mood, sleep, and pain perception.

Vagus nerve. A large nerve that goes from the base of the skull through the trunk of the body, controlling many functions, including the release of the stomach's contents into the small intestine.

APPENDIX 1
INTERNET RESOURCES

The Internet is a rich resource for people seeking information about diabetes. You can educate yourself at your own pace, at times that are convenient for you. Two cautions are in order, however.

First, not everything you find on the Internet will be medically correct or appropriate. Occasionally you will come across information posted by someone who cares more about selling something than about what is appropriate for you. Also, some people put up information that, while it is true as far as their own experience is concerned, is not necessarily true for you. Bring your common sense with you when you go looking around the Internet, evaluate what you read against your own knowledge and experience with your own body, seek the opinions of others you know and respect, and you aren't likely to go wrong.

Second, the Internet is like a living being: It is constantly changing. E-mail lists, newsgroups, and Web sites come and go. Addresses change. The lists that follow are a snapshot taken at a moment in time. If you find addresses that don't work, don't get discouraged. Most will be correct, and with a bit of time and patience, you're almost certain to find what you're looking for, and more that you didn't think of.

E-MAIL LISTS

Electronic mailing lists dedicated to sharing information about diabetes are numerous and varied. When you subscribe to an E-mail list, you begin receiving messages written by other subscribers. If you reply to a message, your reply is sent automatically to every other subscriber. You can also initiate your own message and receive replies from other subscribers. If you don't have your own computer, you might ask at your public library for permission to open an E-mail account and subscribe from there.

Some E-mail lists require that the list manager approve each new subscriber. This requirement is designed to promote subscribers' privacy, not to be exclusive, so don't be shy about asking to be a subscriber. The E-mail addresses given here can be used to apply for a subscription. If the list is open to the public, you will be put on it immediately. If it's a closed list, the request will be sent to the person who manages it. Once you're on the list, you'll be given the address to which to send messages. Most people prefer to read messages for a day or two before replying or asking a question of their own, but that is not a requirement.

Put the welcome message you receive where you can find it; it will come in handy if you want to change your subscription options or leave the list. Don't be shy about joining a list and then leaving it if you find it's not useful to you. You won't insult anyone.

diabetes-subscribe@topica.com
A mailing list for diabetics who want to share information that will help them lead a more healthful and enjoyable life. Not restricted to Type 2. Open to the public without approval.

diabetes2-subscribe@topica.com
For people who have Type 2 diabetes, especially those having trouble controlling their blood sugar. Open to the public without approval.

diabetes-L-subscribe@yahoogroups.com
This is a very active list, intended as a support group for people who have diabetes, care for/about someone with diabetes, or are otherwise interested in living with diabetes.

diabetes_int-subscribe@yahoogroups.com
Support and answers to questions from those who wish to participate in a positive and uplifting debate on this disease, the problems related to it, and different ways to get and keep it under control.

type-2-Diabetes-subscribe@yahoogroups.com
A friendly on-line community for those with Type 2 diabetes. Here you can discuss daily trials and tribulations, what works and doesn't work, as well as find friends.

JewishDiabetes-subscribe@yahoogroups.com
A discussion group about problems and solutions in reconciling the Jewish dietary laws with the nutritional requirements of people with diabetes.

glucolow-subscribe@topica.com
This E-mail list is for individuals with diabetes who are following low-carbohydrate eating plans such as those proposed by Dr. Richard Bernstein, Dr. Robert Atkins, and Drs. Michael and Mary Dan Eades.

DiabetesAndRecovery-subscribe@yahoogroups.com
A discussion group for men and women who have both an eating disorder and an interest in diabetes. Oriented toward the Overeaters Anonymous twelve-step approach.

diabeticos-subscribe@listbot.com
Esta lista de correo electrónico es dedicada a la gente en que habla el español y que tiene la diabetes. (This E-mail list is dedicated to people who speak Spanish and who have diabetes.)

Got-diabetes-subscribe@yahoogroups.com
A friendly and welcoming group, not too much mail; good for people newly diagnosed.

Nowwhat-subscribe@topica.com
A small group, especially welcoming to people new to diabetes. Averages about one message a day, which makes it a good place to start if you don't have much time to spend on-line but want a place to ask questions when you need to.

NEWSGROUPS

Internet newsgroups are much like mailing lists, except that you don't have to send a subscription message and the information sent to newsgroups doesn't come to you as E-mail; you have to go on-line and get it for yourself. Your Internet service provider (ISP) chooses which newsgroups to provide. You may have to ask for a specific newsgroup. The ISP can also help you get set up to receive newsgroups.

alt.support.diabetes and misc.health.diabetes
Both carry general discussions that can be quite lively and informative.

alt.food.diabetic
Recipes and discussions on food.

sci.med.diseases.diabetes
Frequented primarily by physicians, many of whom are willing to answer questions from patients.

WEB SITES

Hundreds of Web sites devoted to diabetes exist to serve you. If you start with the sites listed here and follow the links on them that appeal to you, you won't miss a thing.

http://www.mendosa.com/

Rick Mendosa's Web site contains a wealth of information and links to other sites. It's an ideal place to start your search.

http://www.diabetesmonitor.com/2.htm

Diabetes Monitor is another excellent source of links and information, including detailed information on oral medications, their effects and side effects.

http://www.nlm.nih.gov/medlineplus/diabetes.html
http://www.niddk.nih.gov/health/diabetes/diabetes.htm
http://www.nlm.nih.gov/medlineplus/druginformation.html

These three sites are sponsored by the U.S. National Institutes of Health.

http://www.rxlist.com/

A free, searchable database of more than 4,500 prescription drugs and over-the-counter medications. All the current diabetes drugs are here.

http://www.diabetes.org
The official site of the American Diabetes Association, publishers of *Diabetes Forecast*, a valuable monthly magazine.

http://www.diabetes.ca
The official site of the Canadian Diabetes Association.

http://www.overcomingovereating.com
The official Web site for the Overcoming Overeating program.

http://www.overcomingovereating.com/diabetes.html
For people interested in the Overcoming Overeating method of dealing with compulsive overeating. The book with the same title can be purchased here.

http://vltakaliseji.tripod.com/Vtlakaliseji/id3.html
An Internet Web site for Native Americans.

http://www.glycemicindex.com
An authoritative source of information on the glycemic index of foods, owned by Professor Jennie Brand Miller, author of the leading book on the subject, published in Australia as *The G.I. Factor* and subsequently in the United States and the United Kingdom as *The Glucose Revolution*.

http://www.blackandbrownsugar.com/
Diabetes information specifically meant for people of color.

http://www.alternativediabetes.com
Information about alternative approaches to treating diabetes, including nutritional, herbal, and other strategies.

http://www.hc-sc.gc.ca/hpb/lcdc/publicat/diabet99/d12_e.html
http://www.umanitoba.ca/womens_health/diabmain.htm
http://www.diabeteshealingtrail.ca/traditionalhealing.html
Diabetes information for Canadian aboriginal people.

http://www.overcomingovereating.com
The official Web site for the Overcoming Overeating program.

APPENDIX 2

ORAL DIABETES MEDICATIONS AND THEIR ACTIONS AND SIDE EFFECTS

Managing Type 2 diabetes with diet and exercise is a worthy goal for many people. Oral medication may make sense, particularly in the beginning of your life with diabetes or if diet and exercise are not sufficient to keep your blood sugar under control. But in the long term, it would be a mistake to rely on pills to make up for ignoring the principles of sound blood sugar management.

This appendix is organized by the type of action each medicine performs. The order in which pills are named does not reflect their value or effectiveness.

CLASS: Alpha-Glucosidase Inhibitors

Pills in this class work in the small intestine. They slow the conversion of carbohydrates to glucose, helping to avoid sharp spikes in blood glucose levels. They can be combined with pills in the sulfonylurea or biguanide class, or with injected insulin.

GENERIC NAME: Acarbose

GENERIC AVAILABLE? No

BRAND NAME: Precose in the United States, Prandase in Canada

HOW TO TAKE: With the first bite at each meal

COMMENTS: Acarbose does not cause weight gain or hypoglycemia if it's the only diabetes drug used. If used with other diabetes drugs and hypoglycemia does occur, it can be life threatening, and the patient must use glucose tablets, not table sugar, to overcome this side effect. Correct timing is important; adverse side effects are most commonly gastrointestinal distress: gas, bloating, and diarrhea. Acarbose is not recommended for people with kidney or bowel disorders or nursing mothers; it should not be taken with charcoal (for gas absorption) or digestive enzymes.

GENERIC NAME: Miglitol

GENERIC AVAILABLE? No

BRAND NAME: Glyset

HOW TO TAKE: Same as acarbose

COMMENTS: Same as acarbose

CLASS: BIGUANIDES

Pills in this class improve the body's response to its own insulin. By itself, a biguanide is unlikely to cause hypoglycemia. Biguanides may be combined with sulfonylureas.

GENERIC NAME: Metformin

GENERIC AVAILABLE? No

BRAND NAME: Glucophage in the United States, Glycon in Canada

HOW TO TAKE: Two or three times a day with meals. XR (extended release) version is taken once a day.

COMMENTS: Users sometimes experience nausea, diarrhea, and upset stomach. If any of these symptoms is severe or lasts for more than a few weeks, you should tell your doctor. Rarely, a buildup of lactic acid in the blood can occur, especially in people with impaired kidney or liver function. Lactic acidosis is fatal up to 50 percent of the time. People undergoing x-ray procedures using injectable contrast agents should consult their diabetes doctor because metformin must be discontinued forty-eight hours before the procedure and resumed only after a successful kidney function test. This drug should not be taken by pregnant women.

CLASS: MEGLITINIDES

Pills in this class stimulate the beta cells of the pancreas to release insulin. They are rapidly absorbed and short-acting, concentrating their effects around mealtimes. They may cause hypoglycemia if a meal is skipped. Meglitinides may be combined with metformin.

GENERIC NAME: Repaglinide

GENERIC AVAILABLE? No

BRAND NAME: Prandin in the United States, GlucoNorm in Canada, NovoNorm outside North America

HOW TO TAKE: Immediately before each meal or large snack

COMMENTS: This class of drug is too new to have reliable data on adverse side effects.

GENERIC NAME: NATEGLINIDE
GENERIC AVAILABLE? No
BRAND NAME: Starlix
HOW TO TAKE: Same as Prandin
COMMENTS: Same as Prandin

CLASS: SULFONYLUREAS

These drugs increase insulin release by the beta cells of the pancreas. They also increase cell sensitivity to insulin. They may cause hypoglycemia and may not be a good choice for elderly people or those with kidney disease. Sulfonylureas may be combined with injected insulin or diabetes drugs in other classes.

GENERIC NAME: Glymepride
GENERIC AVAILABLE? No
BRAND NAME: Amaryl
HOW TO TAKE: Once a day

GENERIC NAME: Glyburide
GENERIC AVAILABLE? Yes
BRAND NAME: Diabeta, Glynase, Micronase
HOW TO TAKE: Once or twice a day

GENERIC NAME: Glipizide
GENERIC AVAILABLE? Yes

BRAND NAME: Glucotrol, Glucotrol XL
HOW TO TAKE: Once or twice a day

GENERIC NAME: Acetohexamide
GENERIC AVAILABLE? Yes
BRAND NAME: Dymelor
HOW TO TAKE: Once or twice a day

GENERIC NAME: Chlorpropamide
GENERIC AVAILABLE? Yes
BRAND NAME: Diabinese in the United States; Apo-Chlorpropamide in Canada
HOW TO TAKE: Once a day

GENERIC NAME: Tolazamide
GENERIC AVAILABLE? Yes
BRAND NAME: Tolinase
HOW TO TAKE: Once or twice a day

GENERIC NAME: Tolbutamide
GENERIC AVAILABLE? Yes
BRAND NAME: Orinase
HOW TO TAKE: Two or three times a day

COMMENTS: The brands for which a generic version is available are the first generation of this class of drugs. They have been in use since the 1950s, and their actions and side effects are well known. The second-generation drugs tend to be stronger and have fewer side effects. Orinase is a good choice for people with kidney problems because it doesn't last long in the body. But it is not a good choice for people who often forget to take their pills. Most drugs in this class can cause nausea and flushing in people who drink alcohol. Diabinese is secreted slowly and may not be a good choice for elderly people or those with kidney disease.

WARNING: The unusual shape, color, and size of Amaryl pills are nearly identical to those of Levoxyl, a standard brand of synthetic thyroid hormone. Extreme care must be taken if the patient is prescribed both of these drugs or is in a facility, such as a hospital or nursing home, where both pills are dispensed.

CLASS: Thiazolidinediones

Drugs in this class make cells more sensitive to insulin.

GENERIC NAME: Pioglitazone
GENERIC AVAILABLE? No
BRAND NAME: Actos
HOW TO TAKE: Once a day

GENERIC NAME: Rosiglitazone
GENERIC AVAILABLE? No
BRAND NAME: Avandia
HOW TO TAKE: Once or twice a day
COMMENTS: Thiazolidinediones may be used alone or in combination with other oral diabetes drugs. A blood test for liver function should be done before

starting pills in this class and repeated every two months for the first year. Call your doctor immediately if you experience nausea, vomiting, abdominal pain, fatigue, loss of appetite, or dark urine. All are signs of liver problems. Some drugs in this class may cause fluid retention.

NOTE: Another drug in this class, troglitazone (Rezulin) was withdrawn from the market in 2001 because of problems with liver damage.

APPENDIX 3

BLOOD GLUCOSE MONITORS

With at least thirty blood glucose monitors from which to choose, your best bet for selecting the one that is right for you is to check with your diabetes doctor or diabetes educator. Some diabetes health care teams have special arrangements with manufacturers of certain monitors. They may be able to help you save money. You don't need a prescription for monitors or the supplies required for their use, but you must have one to obtain reimbursement from your insurance company. Don't assume that your insurance covers monitors and supplies; get approval before you buy. To help you make the right decision, you may want to consider these factors.

COST OF MONITOR. Prices vary widely, from about $20 in the United States for a basic monitor to as much as $100 for one with all the bells and whistles. Manufacturers often offer rebates on the price of the monitor; you pay for it, send in a coupon and your receipt, and receive a check for most or all of the purchase price. They can afford to do this because the real cost of monitoring your blood sugars is in the supplies you need to go with the monitor.

COST OF SUPPLIES. The most-needed supplies are two consumable items: test strips and lancets. Test strips collect the blood and are inserted into the monitor to obtain the reading. When you commit to a monitor, you commit to buying the test strips that the monitor uses. Therefore, the cost of the test strips is probably a more important consideration than the initial cost of the monitor. Lancets are the needlelike devices that stick your skin so that you can get blood to test. They fit into a lancing device, so your choice of lancets is determined by your choice of lancing devices. Most often, however, lancing devices are included with monitors, although you can buy lancing supplies separately. For many monitors, you also need a control solution that you use to check the accuracy of the monitor's readings from time to time.

EASE OF USE. Some monitors are easier to use than others. Some require a smaller drop of blood than others.

TEST SITE. Until recently, all glucose monitors required you to stick your fingertip to draw a drop of blood. Some people find this painful; some people have calluses on their fingertips that make it difficult to obtain blood samples. For these individuals, there is a new option: monitors that draw blood from the forearm or other place on the body. Studies have suggested that these monitors are as accurate as finger-stick monitors for fasting blood sugar, but that the forearm monitors give lower results after meals, perhaps because of reduced blood flow in the forearm. Some studies suggest that the accuracy of these monitors is improved by rubbing or tapping the arm before drawing blood.

A new type of meter, recently approved by the U.S. Food and Drug Administration, does away with skin punctures entirely. Designed to be worn on the wrist, it uses an extremely low electric current to measure glucose through the skin every twenty minutes. At present, however, it is very expensive (around $500, plus $60 every two weeks for disposable sensors that wear out after twelve hours) and available only by prescription. It is designed to detect trends and patterns in blood glucose levels and must be used in conjunction with a conventional glucose monitor, not instead of it.

TEST TIME. Monitors can take between a few seconds and a minute to register results. People who are anxious about their results will probably be happier with a fast-registering monitor. Others may not care.

PORTABILITY. Most meters weigh only a few ounces; batteries add a bit of weight but not enough to make this factor very important.

CLEANING AND MAINTENANCE. Monitors require proper care, following the manufacturer's instructions. Few require extensive cleaning or maintenance. You should insist on thorough training in the care and use of your monitor, however. Don't buy one if you can't get taught how to use it.

ACCURACY AND CALIBRATION. Most monitors need to have their accuracy checked periodically. Some use a test solution; some use a calibrator included in each box of test strips; some use both. There's no point in testing your blood glucose if you don't make sure the results are accurate, so you should find out what's required to calibrate your monitor.

BATTERY. Some monitors use AAA batteries; some use smaller ones. A few have a built-in battery, which means that when the battery runs out, you need a new monitor. The warranty on these monitors should match the life of the battery.

WARRANTY. Warranties range from one year to five years. Some warranties are for a certain number of tests.

GLUCOSE RANGE. A monitor should be able to measure low blood sugar as well as high. The widest range available (measured in mg/dl) is 10–600. You probably don't need this wide a range; 40–450 may be sufficient.

RESULTS MEMORY. Most monitors store a number of test results, so that you can recall them for analysis. Some monitors record the date and time of each test. Memories range in size from 20 to 1,000 tests. A few monitors provide a fourteen-day average blood glucose reading. And some have the ability to connect to a personal computer so you can download the results for more permanent storage and, possibly, to send them to your doctor or diabetes educator.

SPECIAL NEEDS. For those with visual impairments, monitors are available that use a synthesized voice to provide instructions and results. Understandably, these are heavier and less portable than most monitors, but they still weigh less than a pound (.45 kg).

APPENDIX 4

ADDITIONAL RESOURCES

ADJUSTING TO CHRONIC ILLNESS

Fennell, Patricia A. *The Chronic Illness Workbook: Strategies and Solutions for Taking Back Your Life.* Oakland, Calif.: New Harbinger, 2001.

DIABETES

Becker, Gretchen E. *The First Year—Type 2 Diabetes: An Essential Guide for the Newly Diagnosed.* New York: Marlowe, 2001.

Bernstein, Richard K. *Dr. Bernstein's Diabetes Solution.* Boston: Little, Brown, 1997.

PM Medical Health News. *Twenty-first Century Complete Medical Guide to Diabetes.* American Diabetes Association CD-ROM, 2002.

Valentine, Virginia, June Beirmann, and Barbara Toohey. *Diabetes Type 2 and What to Do.* Los Angeles: Lowell House, 2000.

DIET AND NUTRITION

Geil, Patti B., and Lea Ann Holzmeister. *One Hundred and One Nutrition Tips for People with Diabetes.* Alexandria, Va.: American Diabetes Association, 1999.

Hirschman, Jane R., and Carol H. Munter. *Overcoming Overeating.* New York: Fawcett, 1989.

Lund, Joanna M., and Janet Meirelles. *The Diabetic's Healthy Exchanges Cookbook.* New York: Perigee, 1996.

Netzer, Corinne T. *The Complete Book of Food Counts.* New York: Dell, 1997.

EXERCISE VIDEOTAPES

Leslie Sandone's In-Home Walking. Charlotte, N.C.: United American Video, 1999.

Stolove, Jodi. *Sit Down and Tone Up.* Delmar, Calif.: Chair Dancing International, 1997.

INSULIN RESISTANCE

Challem, Jack, Burton Berkson, and Melissa Diane Smith. *Syndrome X: The Complete Nutritional Program to Prevent and Reverse Insulin Resistance.* New York: Wiley, 2001.

Romaine, Deborah S., Jennifer B. Marks, and Glenn S. Rothfield. *Syndrome X: Managing Insulin Resistance.* New York: Harper Mass Market Paperbacks, 2000.

Williamson, Miryam Ehrlich. *Blood Sugar Blues: Overcoming the Hidden Dangers of Insulin Resistance.* New York: Walker, 2001.

MOTIVATIONAL SPEAKER

Gary Richards
P.O. Box 129
Westminster, MA 01374
(978) 874-2154

INDEX

A1c
see Hemoglobin A1c test (HbA1c; A1c)
Acceptance
beyond, 52–55
road to, 33–52
Acceptance (stage), 33, 50–52
Acid reflux (heartburn), 30, 31
Activist approach, 57, 58
Adrenal stress hormones, 157
Adult onset diabetes
see Type 2 diabetes
Advice, 172–76
African Americans, 19
Alcohol, 116, 159, 167
Alcoholics, 135
Alcoholics Anonymous (AA), 141, 146, 178
American Diabetes Association (ADA), 56
curriculum by, 61
food pyramid diet, 61, 62, 180
list of recommended foods, 69
Americans with Disabilities Act (ADA), 126
Amino acids, 133
Amputation, 114
Anger (stage), 33, 38–43
Anodyne Therapy System (ATS), 188
Armstrong, Dana, 145
Attitude, 173–76
Autoimmune disease, 31
Autonomic nervous system, 154–55

Bargaining (stage), 33, 43–45
Binge-eating, 2, 136, 139, 142, 145–46

Blood glucose
  see Glucose
Blood sugar, 2, 4
  foods affecting, 72–73, 78, 79, 82–83, 135, 138–39, 150
  monitoring, 129–30, 131
  see also Glucose
Blood sugar levels, 18, 19, 20–21, 27, 30–31, 53, 57
  checking, 29, 37
  in diagnosis stories, 10, 11, 15, 16
  dietary errors and, 65–66
  and erectile dysfunction, 156, 157–58
  exercise and, 89
  fluctuations in, 81–82
  food intake and, 108
  foods raising, 72
  high, 2–10, 28, 66, 150
  high: and sexual dysfunction, 154, 155, 156, 157, 158, 166
  high: and vagus nerve injury, 85, 155
  individual differences in, 171
  keeping within acceptable range, 78, 96
  normal, 66
  oral medications and, 66–67
  reading(s), 9–10, 63
  and sexual dysfunction, 166–67
  working knowledge of, 176
  see also Controlling blood sugar; Fasting blood sugar level; Testing/tests
Blood vessels, 155, 188
  damage to, 4, 110–11, 158
  in genitals, 163
  in penile erection, 154
Body, inborn intelligence about, 177
Body image, 165
Brain, damage to, 87

C-peptide, 86
C-peptide test, 86–87
Canadian Diabetes Association, 12, 20
Capillaries, 110–11, 159
Carbohydrate cravings, 134
Carbohydrates, 32, 43, 71, 72
  for comfort, 116
  diet low in, 27, 62, 69, 74
  excessive intake of, 133
  see also Low-carbohydrate diet
Case stories, 10–16

Overcoming Overeating, 138–48
Cecil Textbook of Medicine, The, 9
Chocolate, 109, 143–44, 147
Cholesterol, 3, 155
Chronic fatigue syndrome, 26–27, 40, 102, 103
Circulation, 110, 155, 166
Circulatory system, 87
Clinical depression, 45, 116
Clitoris, 163
COBRA insurance, 36
Comfort foods, 132, 144, 147, 148
Complications, 36, 124, 178
  dealing with, 110–11
  risk of, 190
  susceptibility to, 87
Compulsive overeating, 2, 46, 105, 132–52
  diet, 149–50
  and lifestyle changes, 151
  negative feelings associated with, 137–38
Congestive heart failure, 37, 69
Controlling blood sugar, 54, 123, 131, 150–51
  diet in, 171
  gastroparesis and, 112–13
  new products and services for, 185–90
  and sexuality, 167, 169
Controlling diabetes, 1, 2, 4, 5, 25, 55, 63, 89, 175–76, 182
  behavior in, 54–55
  key to, 24
  in your hands, 174
Corticosteroids, 31
Council on Aging, 115
Counseling
  for depression, 116

Death(s), 16, 17, 18, 19, 20, 41, 42
  coming to terms with, 33
Dehydration, 28, 30
Dementia, diabetic, 112
Denial (stage), 33, 34–38, 173
Depression, 14, 33, 45, 47, 115–16, 133, 146, 150
  and sexuality, 165–66
Desensitization, 166
Diabeta, 27
Diabetes, 2
  adjusting to, 174–75
  benefits from, 180–84
  coping with, 6–7, 33
  invisible illness, 117–18

patient views of, 180–84
reaction to: men/women differences, 56–57
relationship with, 52–55
uncontrolled, 1, 2, 4, 30
undiagnosed, 111
see also Controlling diabetes; Diabetes management; Learning about diabetes; Type 1 diabetes; Type 2 diabetes
Diabetes education classes, 32, 60–62
Diabetes educator, 32, 35, 51, 59, 60, 79, 178, 189
Diabetes Forecast, 56, 58
Diabetes management, 5–6, 25, 58, 67–68, 131
diet in, 88
effect on family, 122
exercise in, 27, 88–89, 91–92
goal of, 78
grief stages in, 33
hurdles in, 97–131
integrating with life outside home, 125–26
knowledge in, 176–80
weight loss in, 150
Diabetes management program, 188–89
Diabetic coma, 31
Diabetic neuropathy *see* Neuropathy
Diagnosis, 6, 8–10, 28, 29, 31–32, 77
feelings about, 173
lack of, 25–27
reactions to, 17–23, 33
reactions to: anger, 38–43
reactions to: bargaining, 43–45
reactions to: denial, 34–38
reactions to: grief, 45–50
Diagnosis stories, 8, 10–16
Diet, 1, 2, 24, 32, 52–53, 123–24
ADA, 61, 62, 180
in diabetes management, 88
diabetic, 24, 149–50
and exercise, 93–94, 104
in glucose management, 190
and health, 69–70
high-carbohydrate, 32, 61, 70
individual differences, 171

low–carbohydrate, 27, 33, 62, 74, 69, 171, 180
and medication, 76
Dietary errors, consequences of, 65–66
Dietary restriction, 143, 146
Dietician, 28, 31, 32, 43, 70, 98, 108
Dieting, 29, 46, 140, 141, 143
leads to overeating, 138
Digestive disorders, 85
Dizziness, 15, 66
Doctors, 7, 25–33, 136, 178
anger at, 40, 42–43
failure to diagnose, 10
instructions to patients, 79
problems with, 97–102
questioning, 179
women and, 165–66
Dr. Bernstein's Diabetes Solution, 33
Drugs
see Medications

Eating, 75, 131
emotional, 148
frequency of, 73–74
out of control, 134
reasons for, 115–16
on regular schedule, 66, 67
relearning, 105–10
variability in, 117–19
Eating disorder(s), 26
Eating right, 63–77
individual variation in, 70
Electrocardiogram (EKG), 85
Emotional eating, 148
Emotions, 81–82, 115
in sexual stimulation, 156
Endocrinologist, 30, 36, 38, 59, 98, 101
Endorphins, 94, 116
Endothelium, 155, 156
Energy, 2, 9, 10, 53
decrease in, 133
exercise and, 94, 103
Erectile dysfunction, 153, 154–63
overcoming, 159–62
Exercise, 1, 24, 27–28, 32, 53, 61, 87–96, 131, 181
benefits from, 94–95
and depression, 116
in diabetes management, 27, 88–89, 91–92
gastroparesis and, 113
in glucose management, 190

obstacles to, 102–5
and penile erection, 159

Family, 119, 120–21, 122, 124, 172
Family history, 8, 18, 22, 36, 40, 45, 50–51
Fasting blood sugar level, 21, 22, 62, 92
Fasting blood sugar test, 9–10, 77
Fatigue (symptom), 9, 11, 14, 18, 66, 111
at work, 127
see also Chronic fatigue syndrome
Fear, 174, 178
Fiber supplement, 76
Fibromyalgia, 30
Finger stick, 25–26, 80–81
Finger-stick monitor, 81
Food(s), 46
affecting blood sugar, 72–73, 78, 79, 82–83, 135, 138–39, 150
causing blood sugar spikes, 170
changing how you think about, 136–38
controlling amount of, 107
effects on blood sugar, 53, 137, 151
freedom to choose, 144
making peace with, 148–52
relationship with, 134, 141, 142
response to distress, 132–33, 134
as trigger, 176
Food and Drug Administration, 185–86
Food choices, 65, 68
Food cravings, 108, 133
carbohydrates, 134
sweets, 109–10, 147
Food intake, 85
and blood sugar levels, 108, 151
coordinated with medicine intake, 67
keeping track of, 150–51
restricting, 137, 142
Food pyramid, 32, 61, 62
Foot clinics, 114–15
Foot problems, 110, 114–15
Foreplay, 160, 162
Friends, 120, 121–23, 172

Gastroparesis, 111–14
Genetic tendency, 8
Genital engorgement, 163
Genitals
malfunction of female, 163

Gestational diabetes, 1, 51
Ghrelin, 188
Glucagon-like-peptide-1 (GLP-1), 187–88
Glucose, 2
  foods turn into, 72
  measuring, 16, 87
  stored as fat, 3
  stored for energy, 66
  see also Blood sugar levels
Glucose control, 46–47
Glucose meter(s)/monitor(s), 12, 28, 31, 32, 36, 63, 71, 75, 78, 81, 101–2, 119, 130, 149, 176, 186, 190
  new, 185–86, 213–17
Glucose test, 11, 62, 78–83
Glucose tolerance test, 27, 77–78
Glycemic index, 72, 73
Glycogen, 66, 171
God, 44–45
Grief
  stages of, 33–52, 115

Health
  diet and, 69–70
Health care professionals, 167, 190
  mixed messages from, 25
Health care team, 102
Health clubs, 90
Health insurance, 36–37, 61, 188–89
Health maintenance organizations (HMOs), 101
  courses offered by, 34
  diabetes classes, 60–61, 62
Heart, damage to, 87
Heart attack, 29, 155
Heart disease, 3
Heart rate, 86
Hemoglobin (Hb), 84
Hemoglobin A1c test (HbA1c; A1c), 83–85, 87, 91–92, 106, 123
  decreasing, 188, 190
  kits for testing at home, 186
Heredity, 40, 65, 170
High blood pressure, 3, 156, 158
Hirschman, Jane, 145
Hospitals
  diabetes classes, 60–61, 32
  diabetes support groups, 179, 180
Hunger, 136, 148
  causes of, 136
Hyperglycemia, 9
Hypoglycemia, 66, 71, 86, 98–99, 100, 171

reactive, 15
symptoms, 111
Hypoglycemic episodes, 113

Ice cream, 76–77, 109–10
Immune system, 2–3
Impotence, 153
Individual differences, 7, 170–72
Infection, 81, 110, 114
Information
getting, 36, 58–63
sources, 108, 219–21
Information packet, 59
Inner child, reconnecting with, 152
Insomnia, 133
Insulin, 2, 3, 73, 78
and alcohol, 159
and blood glucose test, 79–80, 82
body's response to, 81–82
exercise and sensitivity to, 92–93, 94, 159
function of, 66
high, 134
imbalance with serotonin, 136
insufficient, 46
new methods for delivery of, 186–87
and nitric oxide, 156
release by pancreas, 26
synthetic, 53
too much, 133
Insulin injections, 3, 24, 29, 31, 61, 112–13, 122
Insulin resistance, 3, 4, 46, 86–87
cause of Type 2 diabetes, 13, 155
and compulsive overeating, 134
decreasing, 103
in erectile dysfunction, 155–56
exercise as weapon against, 88–89
Intercourse, 164, 168
Internet, 9, 35, 58–60, 62, 76, 100, 101, 110, 139
access to, 57
reliability of information, 59, 108
resources, 197–204
support groups, 179–80
Interpersonal relationships, 116–25
Interstitial fluid, 185, 189
Irregular heartbeat, 11, 37, 69

Jenkins, David, 72
Juvenile diabetes
see Type 1 diabetes

Kennedy, John F., 102
Ketoacidosis, 30
Kidneys, damage to, 87, 151
Knowledge, 57, 61–62
  as power, 176–80
Kubler–Ross, Elizabeth, 33, 34, 43, 45, 50

Lean diabetics, 3
Learning about diabetes, 32–33, 56–96, 101, 108, 172, 176–80
Libido, 156
  loss of, 164
Library(ies), 57, 180
Life changes, 174, 175, 181, 184
Lifestyle, 36, 39, 55, 128
  changes in, 151
  healthy, 57
  sedentary, 4
Lifestyle choices, 16, 190
Liver, 66
Liver function test, 99
Low-carbohydrate diet, 27, 33, 62, 69, 74, 171, 180

Managing diabetes
  see Diabetes management
Meal planning, 6, 61, 65, 73, 74
Meals
  size and frequency, 74
Medical knowledge, 57
Medical team, 98
Medications, 2, 25, 26, 27, 28, 29, 30, 54, 112, 113, 151
  and alcohol, 159
  for depression, 116
  and erectile dysfunction, 158
  insulin-stimulating, 32–33
  masking symptoms, 12–13
  new, 187
  and sexual dysfunction, 167
  see also Oral medications
Men
  reaction to diabetes, 56–57, 58
  sexual dysfunction, 153–63, 166
Menstrual period, 82
Mental confusion, 66, 111
Mental health professionals, 138
Metabolism, 94, 176
Mind
  reprogramming, 137
  in sexual stimulation, 156

Monitoring blood sugar, 129–30, 131
  compulsive, 148–49
  devices for, 187
  see also Glucose meter(s)/monitor(s)
Morbid obesity, 26
Mortality, diagnosis as reminder of, 47–49
Motivation, 115
  for exercise, 92–93
MUSE system, 162

Native Americans, 13, 43, 51, 170
Nerves
  circulation to, 188
  damage to, 4, 14, 110, 111, 166–67
  in genitals, 163
  in penile erection, 154
Neuropathy, 4, 86, 98, 110, 114, 150
  effect on genitals, 163–64
  new treatment for, 188
  in vagus nerve, 111, 112, 155, 161
Newton, Isaac, 87–88
Nitrates, 160
Nitric oxide, 155–56, 160, 163
  increasing supply of, 188
Nitroglycerine, 160
Nutritional supplements, 76
Nutritionist, 59, 60, 70, 101–2, 136, 178

Obesity, 3, 4, 8, 138
  morbid, 26
On Death and Dying (Kubler-Ross), 33
Ophthalmologist, 98
Oral medications, 2, 24, 61, 62, 73, 76, 205–11
  and blood sugar levels, 66–67
  individual choices in, 171–72
  wrong, 99–100
  see also Medications
Orgasm, 162, 168
Overcoming Overeating (OO), 46, 136–37, 138–45
  case stories, 138–48
Overeaters Anonymous (OA), 136, 141, 142

Pancreas, 2, 66, 86, 159
  producing insufficient insulin, 3, 46
Papaverine, 162
Passive approach, 57
Patient role, 189–90
Penile constriction ring, 161

Penile erection, 154–55
Penile prostheses, 161–62
Peripheral circulation, damage to, 150–51
Peripheral vascular disease, 155
Phentolamine, 162
Podiatrist, 98
Portion size, 107
Predisposition to diabetes, 51
Primary care practitioner, 98
Products and services, new, 185–90
Prostaglandin, 162
Proteins, 133
Psychiatrist, 116
Psychological counselor(s), 136, 165
Psychological factors, 134, 140, 183–84

R-point, 86
R-to-R interval study, 85–86, 113–14
Range-of-motion exercise, 103
Reactive hypoglycemia, 15
Reading labels, 10, 30, 107, 125
Rebound bingeing, 142, 143
Record keeping, 61, 149, 176, 181
Recreational eating, 64, 106
Resources, 215–21
Restaurant eating, 68, 133
Retrograde ejaculation, 162–63
Rocking, 102–3

Seasons, change of, 82
Self-advocacy, 7
Self-diagnosis, 12, 23, 37
Serotonin, 133
  imbalance with insulin, 136
Sex, importance of, 167–69
Sex therapists, 168
Sexual arousal, 163–64, 167
Sexual dysfunction, 7, 83, 111, 153–69
Sexual stimulation, 156–57, 160
Sildenafil
  see Viagra
Situational depression, 45, 115
  counseling for, 116
Smoking, 158
Snacks, 128–29
Sneaking food, 123
Social situations, 121, 122–23

Specialists, 98, 101
Spikes, 72, 73, 76
  avoiding foods causing, 114
  controlling, 174
  exercise and, 93
  foods causing, 170
Spontaneity, loss of, 6, 47, 181
Standing up for yourself, 97–102
"Stinking thinking," 137, 138
Stress, 14, 124, 127–28, 146
  and fluctuations in blood sugar levels, 81–82
  and serotonin, 133
  as trigger, 176
Stroke, 3, 155
Sugar
  in diet, 68
Support, 104–5
Support groups, 5, 105, 179–80
Sweets, 29, 64, 150
  for comforting, 40–41
  cravings, 109–10, 147
Symptoms, 6, 8, 9, 14, 15, 18, 66
  of gastroparesis, 111
  hypoglycemic, 111
  masked by medications, 12–13
Taking responsibility for your diabetes, 98, 117, 125, 178, 190
Telemedicine, 189
Terminal illness
  coping strategies in, 33
Testing/tests, 6, 24, 35, 61, 63, 75, 76, 77–87, 138–39, 150, 159, 177, 181
  amount of, 149
  frequency, 24, 71, 79–80, 83
  knowledge obtained from, 177
  in public, 129–30
Testosterone, 156
Thirst (symptom), 9, 10, 11, 13, 14, 18, 19
Time frames, eating within, 108–9
Tobacco, 158
  and sexual dysfunction, 167
Travel, 67–68
Treatment plan, 57, 189
Treats, 29, 76
Trigger(s), 135, 136, 176
Twelve-step groups, 136, 137, 141
Type 1 diabetes, 2–3, 98
  C-peptide test, 86, 87
Type 2 diabetes, 1, 2, 3–6, 88, 156

adjusting to life with, 24–55
hurdles in managing, 97–131
increase in, 3–4, 185
individual differences, 170–72
insulin resistance as cause of, 13, 155
positive effect of, 5
receiving diagnosis of, 17–23
and sexual dysfunction, 153–54

University of Massachusetts in Amherst, 88–89
Urinary tract infections, 167
Urination, frequent (symptom), 9, 10, 11, 13, 14, 18, 19
Urine sample, 25, 77
Urologist, 162, 163
U.S. Centers for Disease Control, 3–4

Vacuum erection device, 160–61
Vaginal dryness, 164, 167
Vaginal lubricants, 164
Vaginal sphincter, 164
Vaginal wall, 163
Vaginal yeast infections (symptom), 11–12, 167
Vaginitis, 167
Vagus nerve, 86
damage to, 85, 155
neuropathy in, 111, 112
and penile erection, 154–55
Value judgments, 134–35, 137, 144, 149, 150
Viagra, 160, 161, 163
Vision
blurry (symptom), 13, 53, 66
damage to, 87, 150
Vulva, 163

Walking, 90, 95
Water exercise, 103
Weight
and work, 128
Weight gain, 140, 141, 143, 146
Weight loss, 19, 37, 150
exercise and, 94, 95
obstacles to, 102–5
Weight loss (symptom), 11–12, 14

Women
  reaction to diabetes, 56–57
  sexual dysfunction, 154, 163–67
Work, 121, 125–29
Writing things down, 115–16